365

DAILY EXERCISES

Microworkouts for Busy People

2021

N. Rey | darebee.com

First Printing, 2021.
ISBN 13: 978-1-84481-177-9
ISBN 10: 1-84481-177-8

Warning and Disclaimer
Although every precaution has been taken to verify the accuracy of the information contained herein, the author and publisher assume no responsibility for any errors or omissions. No liability is assumed for damage or injury that may result from the use of information contained within.

Introduction

We are all busy. There are days when life becomes complicated and time is not on our side. That doesn't mean that fitness has to stop. Fitness, really, is an investment in time and effort that we make to ensure the quality of life of our own older, future self.

This means that when we have less time and energy to devote to it we still need to find a way to maintain the gains we have made. This is where microworkouts and Daily Exercises come in.

Daily Exercises are a short, snappy exercise you do once a day, each day of the week. It is designed to activate your cardiovascular system and challenge as many muscle groups and tendons as possible.

Each exercise is relatively easy to perform. some are very short. In their totality however, 365 of them represent a significant commitment to fitness that over the course of a year delivers visible results. Because each Daily Dare is designed to challenge you a little without tiring you out you can do one each day even if you're going to exercise hard at some point later. On your busiest day when you have no time to do anything else you will still feel strong, healthy and better able to cope with stress.

There are 365 Daily Exercises in this book. One for each day of the year. Ideally you start at the first one, complete it, tick the box next to it on the page and keep track of where you are in the book, this way. If you're not sure how to do a particular exercise you can check out the Darebee exercise library at the link below:

Video How-Tos / Library:
https://darebee.com/video

1

50 Jumping Jacks

Do jumping jacks until you hit 50 in total. Split into manageable sets.

Extra Credit: in one go

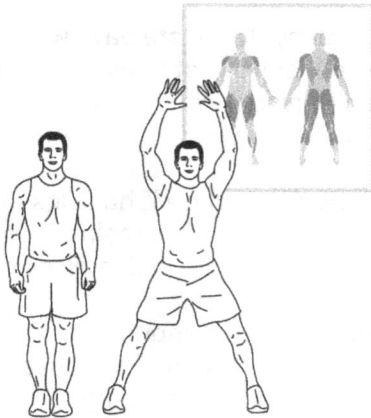

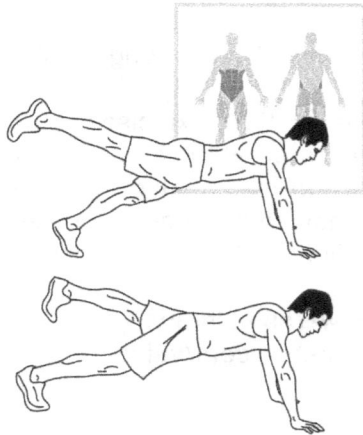

2

6 Raised Leg Push-Ups

Get into a plank position and raise your left leg, lower yourself down and then push yourself up - 6 times in total. Switch legs every time. Split into manageable sets.

Extra Credit: in one go

3

30 Reverse Angels

Lie on the floor face down, arms
extended in front of you. Bring your
arms to your sides as illustrated 30
times in total. Split into manageable
sets.

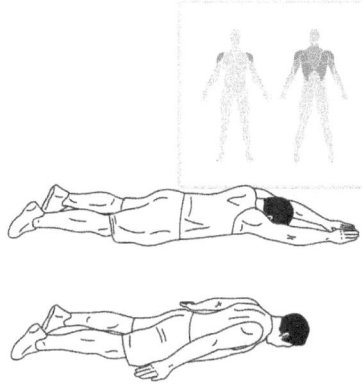

Extra Credit: in one go

4

20 Reverse Crunches

Lie down on the floor, legs bent
at roughly 90 degrees. Roll your
lower body up towards your chest
as illustrated - 20 times in total. Split
into manageable sets.

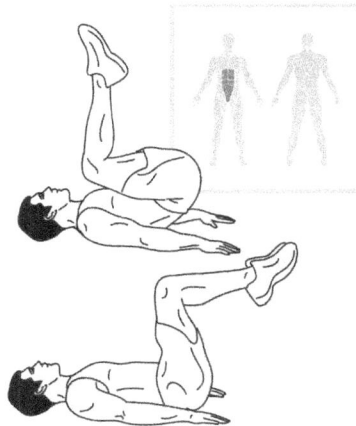

Extra Credit: in one go

30 Seconds One-Arm Plank

Hold a one-arm plank for 30 seconds in total. Split into manageable sets. Switch arms halfway through.

Extra Credit: in one go

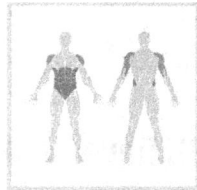

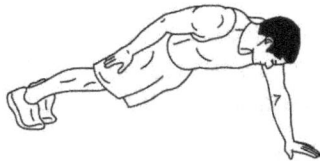

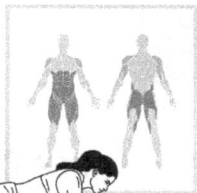

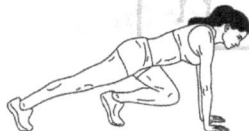

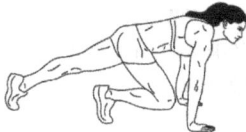

60 Climbers

Get down into a plank. Begin to climb on the spot, as fast as you can, until you hit 60 reps in total (30 per leg). Split into manageable sets.

Extra Credit: in one go

7

40 Lunge Step-Ups

Start from a lunge and step up 40
times in total, 20 times per side
(complete one side first, then the
other). Split into manageable sets.

Extra Credit: in one go

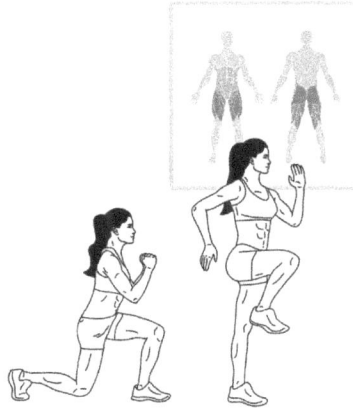

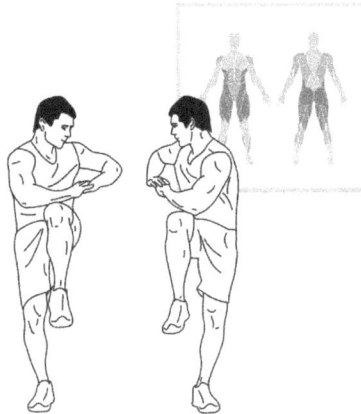

8

40 March Twists

March on the spot while twisting so
your opposite elbow touches your
opposite knee, as illustrated - 40
times in total.

Extra Credit: in one go

9

2 Minutes Hops on the Spot

Set a timer and bounce on the spot (two feet) for 2 minutes in total. Try to keep pauses to a minimum.

Extra Credit: non-stop

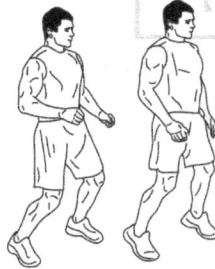

10

50 Squats

Do squats until you hit 50 in total. Split into manageabe sets - as fewer as possible.

Extra Credit: in one go

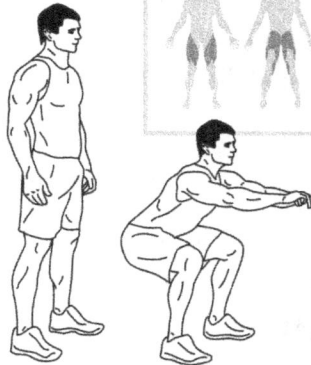

11

20 Plank Jacks

Do squats until you hit 20 in total.
Split into manageabe sets - as fewer
as possible.

Extra Credit: in one go

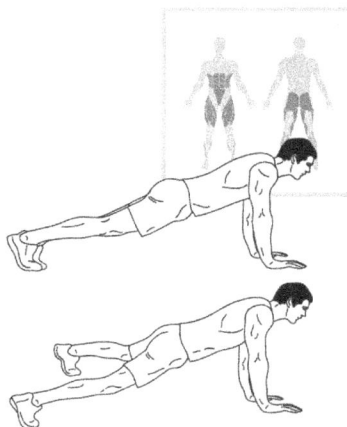

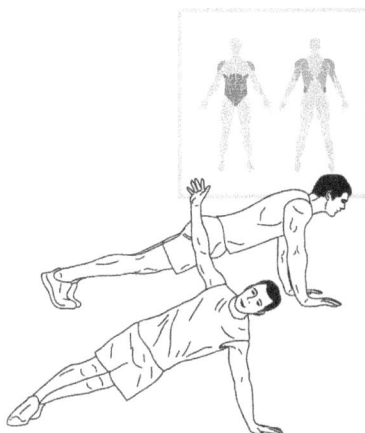

12

20 Plank Rotations

Get into a plank and do rotations as
illustrated until you hit 20 in total.
Split into manageable sets.

Extra Credit: in one go

13

2 Minutes Sitting Punches

Sit down, body at roughly 45 degrees and throw punches for 2 minutes in total. Split into manageable sets.

Extra Credit: non-stop

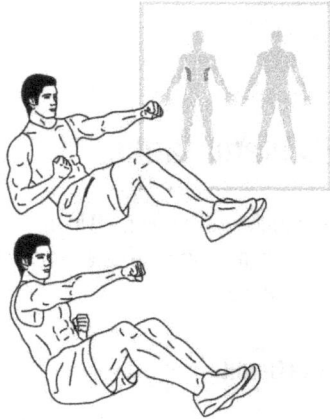

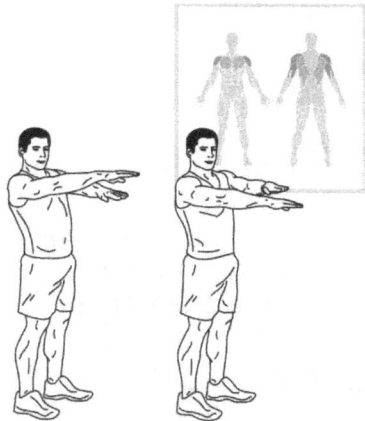

14

2 Minutes Arm Scissors

Set a timer and do arm scissors as fast as you can for 2 minutes in total. Split into manageable sets.

Extra Credit: non-stop

15

10 Basic Burpees With a Jump

Do basic burpees with a jump (no push-up) as fast as you can until you hit 10 in total. Split into manageable sets.

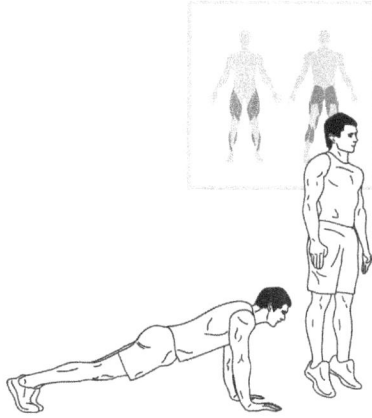

Extra Credit: in one go

16

40 Knee In & Twists

Sit down on the floor, legs extended in front of you. Bring your knees in while twisting them to your side. Repeat 40 times in total. Split into manageable sets.

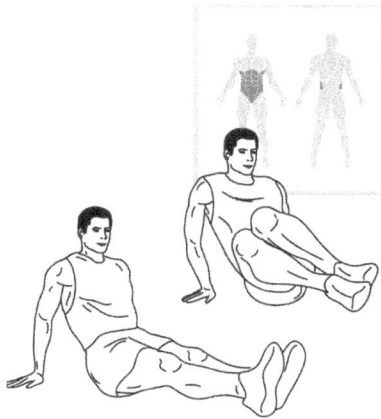

Extra Credit: in one go

60 Seconds Jumping Ts

Set a timer and do jumping Ts for
60 seconds in total.
Split into manageable sets.

Extra Credit: non-stop

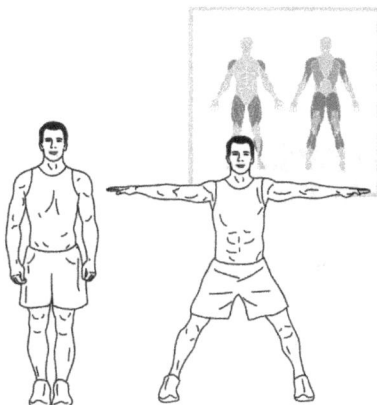

30 Scissors

Lie down, raise your legs at roughly
30 degrees off the floor and do
scissors in the air until you hit 30
reps, cross over & under = 2 reps.

Extra Credit: in one go

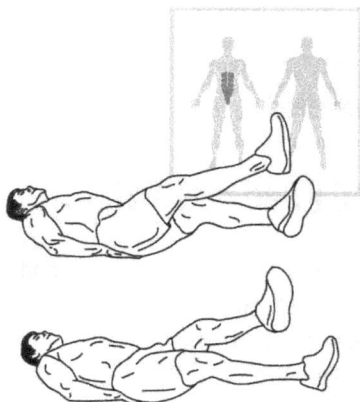

19

30 Seconds High Knees

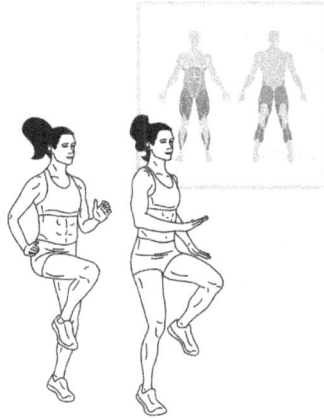

Set a timer and do high knees (sprint on the spot) for 30 seconds in total. Split into manageable sets.

Extra Credit: non-stop

20

10 Up & Down Planks

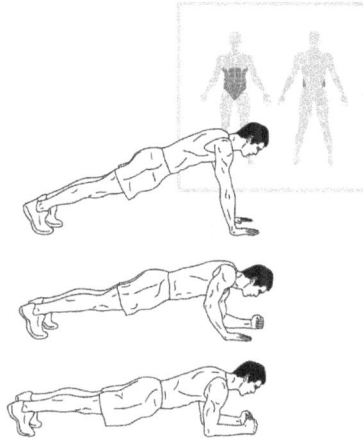

Lower yourself from a plank into an elbow plank - 10 times in total. All the way down and all the way up is 1 rep. Split into manageable sets.

Extra Credit: in one go,

keep the plank

60 Side Leg Raises

Raise your right leg to your side at 90 degrees until you hit 30 reps; change legs and do another 30, 60 in total. You can hold on to something.

Extra Credit: 30/30 in one go

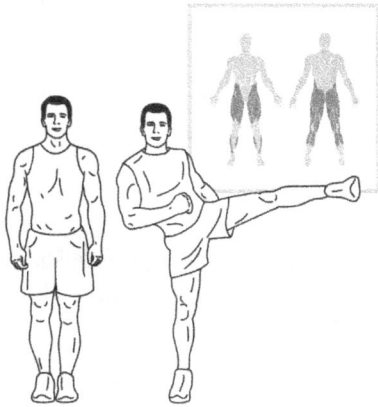

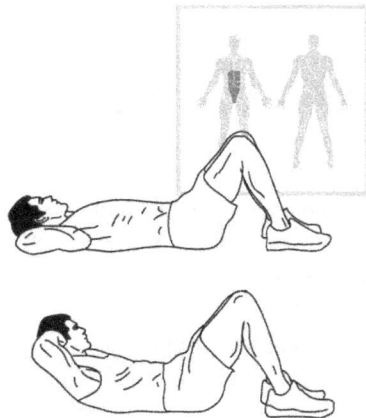

50 Crunches

Lie down on the floor (place something soft under you) until you hit 50 in total.

Extra Credit: in one go

23

10 Plank Walk-Outs

Walk out into a plank, as illustrated, until you hit 10 in total. Split into manageable sets.

Extra Credit: in one go

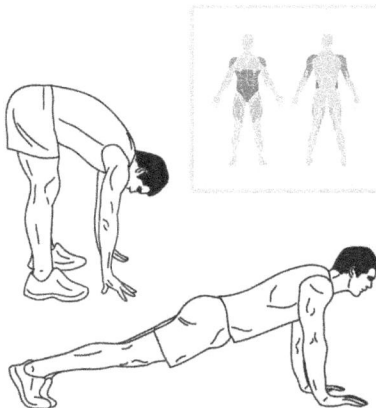

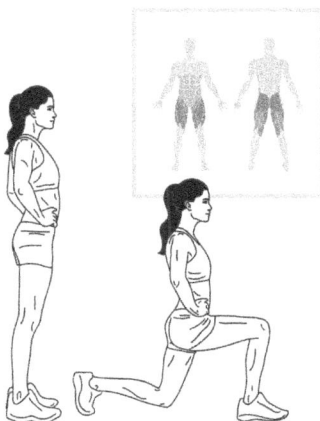

24

30 Forward Lunges

Step into a forward lunge 30 times in total. Split into manageable sets.

Extra Credit: in one go

25

60 Seconds Clench / Unclench

Set a timer then clench and unclench your hands as fast as you can for 60 seconds in total. Split into manageable sets.

Extra Credit: non-stop

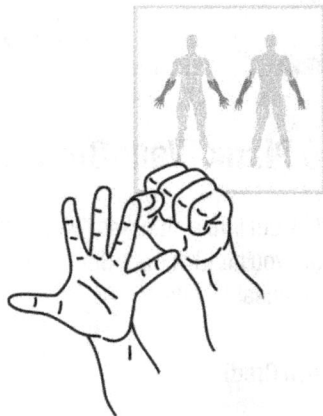

26

20 Bridge Taps

Lie down, raise your hips up and tap the floor over your head. Repeat 20 times in total. Split into manageable sets.

Extra Credit: in one go

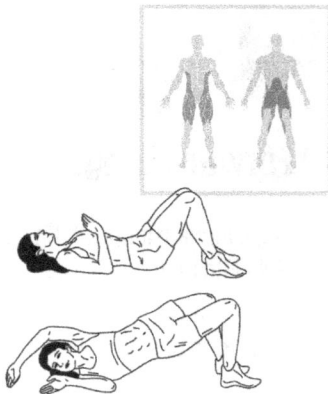

60 Standing Shoulder Taps

Tap your shoulders and raise your arms up reaching for the ceiling - 60 times in total. Split into manageable sets.

Extra Credit: in one go

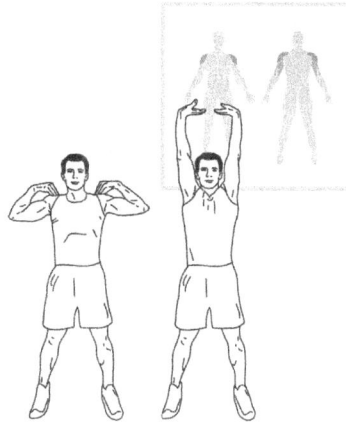

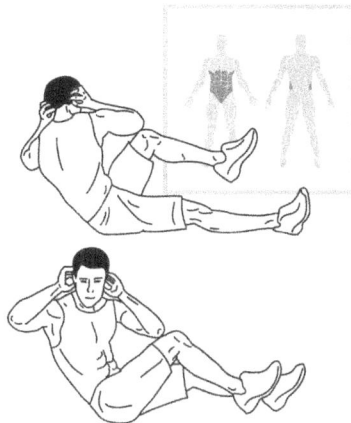

30 Knee-to-Elbow Crunches

Get on the floor, place your hands behind your head and bring the opposite knee to opposite elbow 30 times in total.

Extra Credit: in one go

60 Seconds Wall-Sit

Set a timer and sit against the wall as illustrated. Hold it for 60 seconds in total. Split into manageable sets.

Extra Credit: in one go

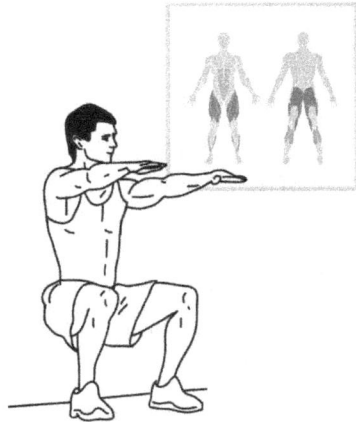

100 Overhead Punches

Do overhead punches, 50 with the right arm, 50 with the left arm, 100 times in total. Complete one side first before starting on the other. Split into manageable sets.

Extra Credit: 100/100, in one go

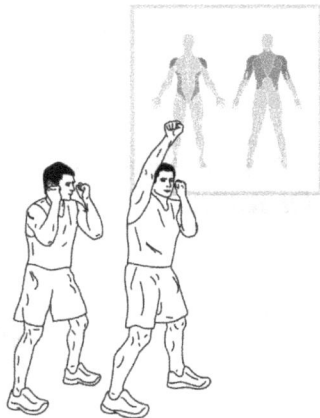

31

60 Seconds Plank Punches

Set a timer and get into a plank. Throw punches as fast as you can for 60 seconds in total. Split into manageable sets.

Extra Credit: non-stop

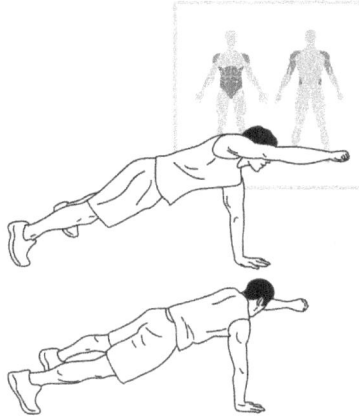

32

30 Side Bridges

Get into a side elbow plank, lower your hips to the floor and come up again - 30 times in total; 15 per side. Split into manageable sets.

Extra Credit: 15/15 in one go

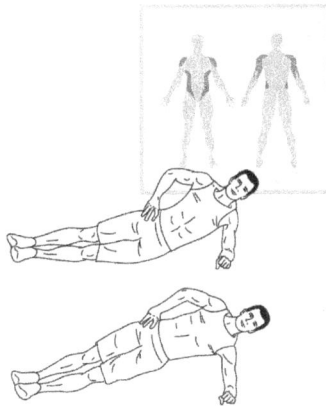

33

5 Clapping Push-Ups

Get on the floor and do push-ups,
clap every time as you come up -
5 in total. Split into manageable sets.

Extra Credit: in one go

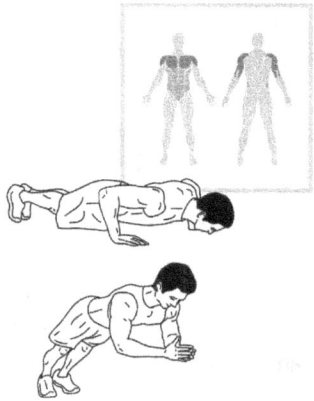

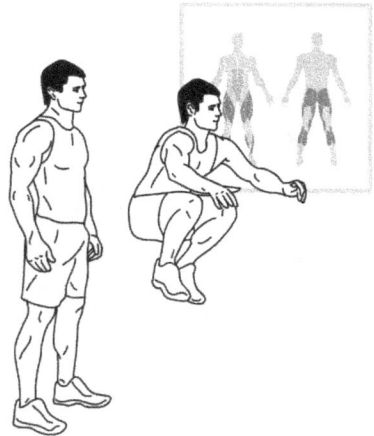

34

5 Jump Knee Tucks

Jump up bringing your knees to your
chest - 5 times in total.
Split into manageable sets.

Extra Credit: in one go

35

60 Seconds Butt Kicks

Set a timer and do butt kicks for 60 seconds in total. Split into manageable sets.

Extra Credit: non-stop

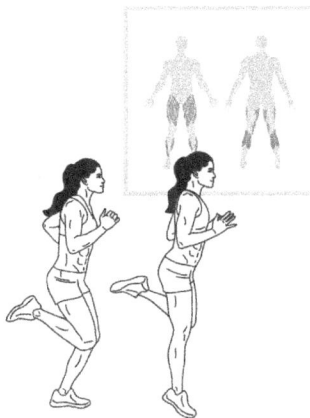

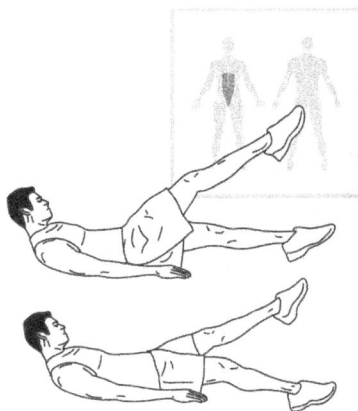

36

30 Seconds Flutter Kicks

Set a timer and do flutter kicks as fast as you can for 30 seconds in total. Split into manageable sets.

Extra Credit: non-stop

37

60 Bicep Extensions

Bring your arms to your ears and unroll them out palm outwards, as illustrated, 60 times in total. Split into manageable sets.

Extra Credit: in one go

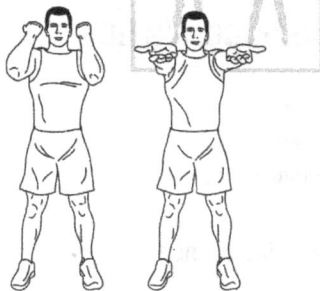

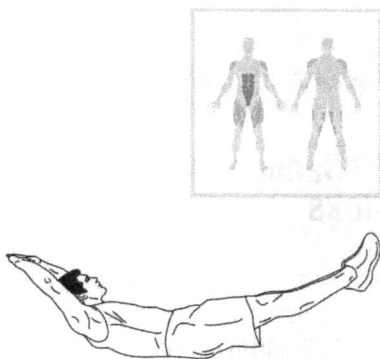

38

30 Seconds Hollow Hold

Stretch out, raise your arms and legs off the floor as illustrated. Hold it for 30 seconds in total. Split into manageable sets.

Extra Credit: in one go

40 Seal Jacks

Start with your arms raised to your sides, legs wide then jump in, bringing your hands together. Repeat 40 times in total.

Extra Credit: in one go

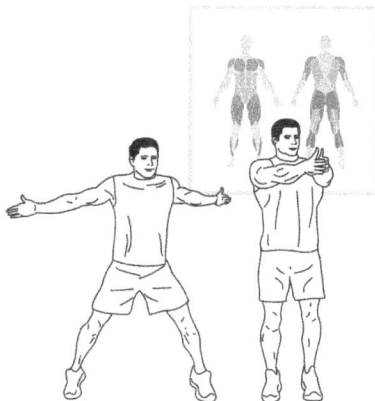

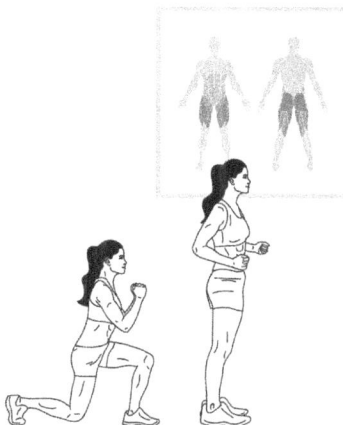

20 Reverse Lunges

Step back into a lunge - 20 times in total. Split into manageable sets.

Extra Credit: in one go

41

20 Hop Heel Clicks

Hop up and click your heels - 20 times in total. Split into manageable sets.

Extra Credit: in one go

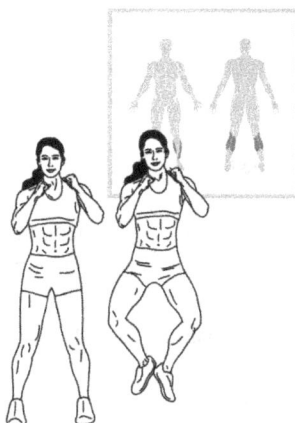

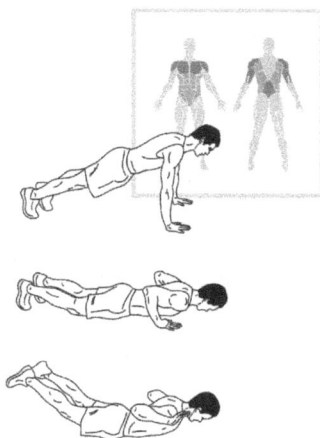

42

10 Sky Diver Push-Ups

Get into a plank position and drop down so your chest rests on the floor, raise your arms up as illustrated. Push back up. repeat 10 times in total.

Extra Credit: in one go

43

50 Calf Raises

Stand up straight, arms behind your
back and raise up onto your toes
- 50 times in total. Split into
manageable sets.

Extra Credit: in one go

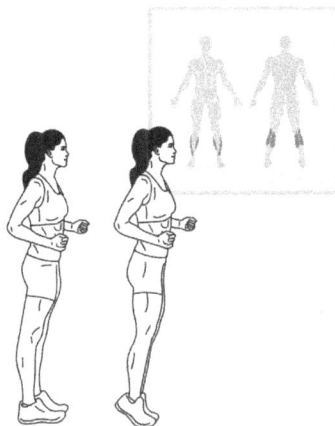

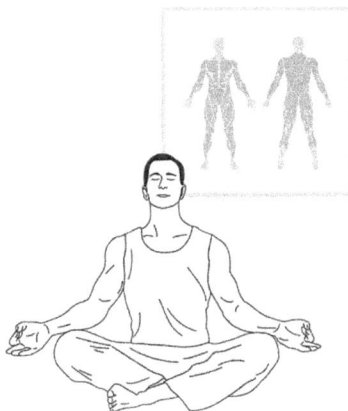

44

2 Minutes Meditation

Set a timer and meditate for 2
minutes in total. Relax. Keep cool.
Breathe.

Extra Credit: in one go

45

20 Seagulls

Get into an elbow plank, stretch your hand in front of you and move it to the side. Repeat until you hit 20 reps in total. Split into manageable sets.

Extra Credit: in one go

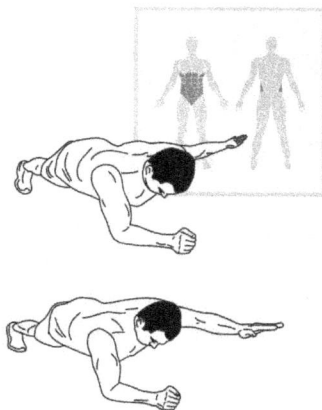

46

60 Seconds Raised Arm Circles

Set a timer, raise your arms up shoulder height and rotate them for 60 seconds in total. Split into manageable sets.

Extra Credit: non-stop

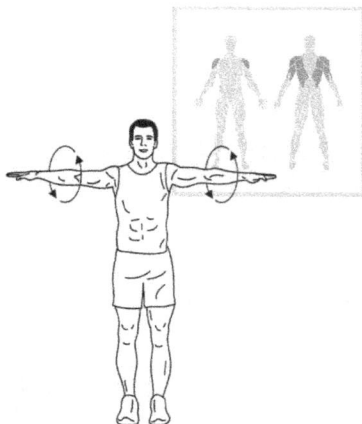

47

30 Seconds Reverse Plank Hold

Get into a reverse plank position
as illustrated - and hold it for 30
seconds in total.
Split into manageable sets.

Extra Credit: in one go

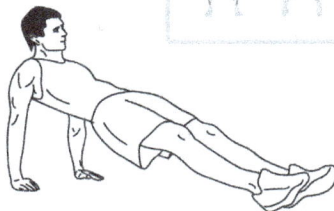

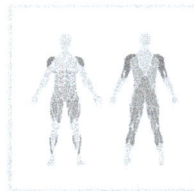

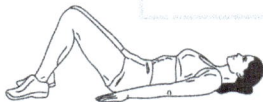

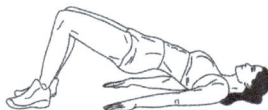

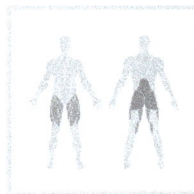

48

30 Bridges

Lie down, knees bent as illustrated
and raise your hips off the floor
= 30 times in total. Split into manageable sets.

Extra Credit: in one go

49

60 Seconds Skiers

Set a timer and do skiers, as illustrated for 60 seconds in total. Split into manageable sets.

Extra Credit: in one go

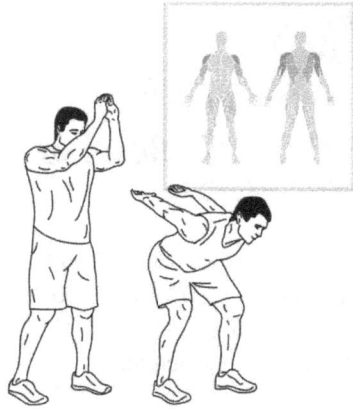

50

4 Minutes Raised Arms Hold

Set a timer and hold arms raised in front of you at shoulder height for 4 minutes in total. Split into manageable sets.

Extra Credit: in one go,

keep arms up

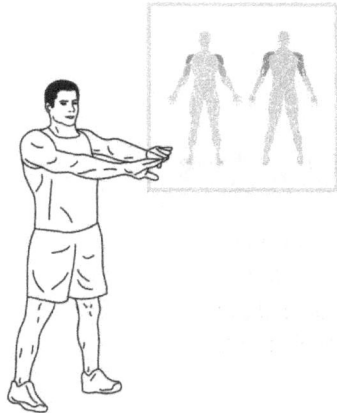

40 Knee Crunches

Lie down on the floor, bring your knees up and lean forward until your elbows and knees touch - 40 times in total. Split into manageable sets.

Extra Credit: in one go

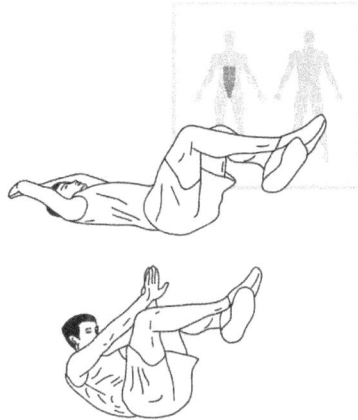

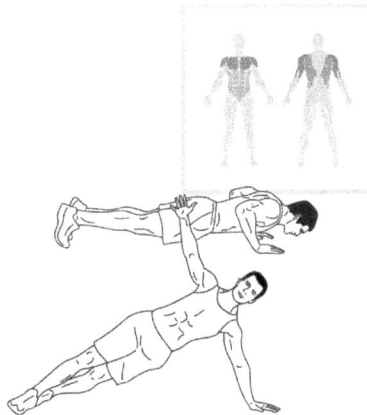

10 Push-Up
With Rotations

Get on the floor and lower yourself into a push-up, come up and turn into a side plank - 10 times in total; split into manageable sets.

Extra Credit: in one go

30 Cross Reach Sit-Ups

Lie down on the floor and raise one arm towards the ceiling. Sit-up and reach with opposite arm towards opposite foot- 30 times in total. Split into manageable sets.

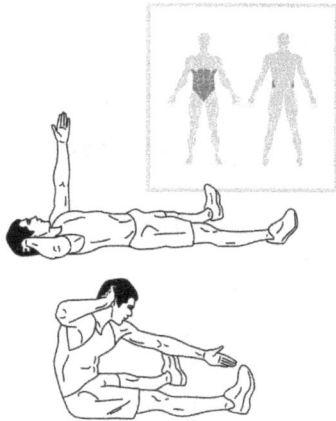

Extra Credit: in one go

60 W-Arm Extensions

Raise your arms up and then lower them down until your elbows are at shoulder level - as illustrated. Repeat 60 times in total. Split into manageable sets.

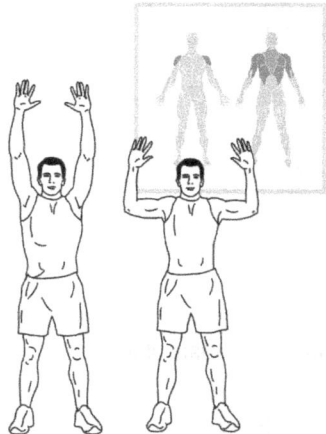

Extra Credit: in one go

30 Seconds Squat Hold

Lower yourself into a squat (your glutes should be parallel to the floor) and hold it for 30 seconds in total. Split into manageable sets.

Extra Credit: in one go

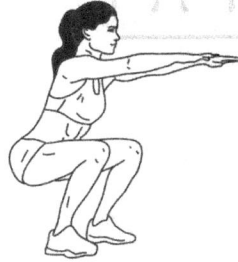

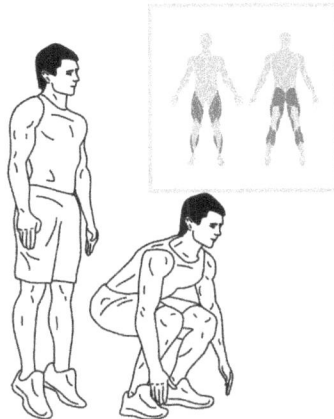

10 Jump Squats

Do jump squats until you hit 10 in total. Split into manageable sets.

Extra Credit: in one go

57

100 Squat Hold Punches

Lower yourself into a squat, hold it and throw punches until you hit 100 punches in total.
Split into manageable sets.

Extra Credit: in one go

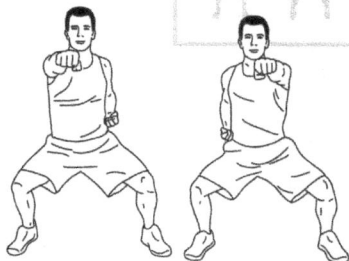

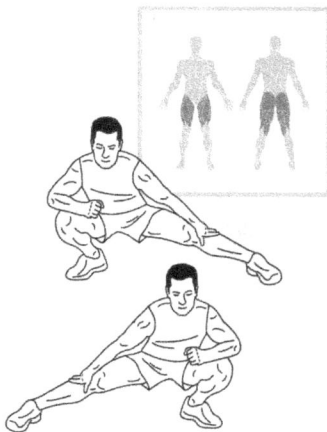

58

30 Side-To-Side Lunges

Get into a deep side lunge position and shift your body to the other side without standing up, 30 times in total. Split into manageable sets.

Extra Credit: in one go

59

60 Seconds Calf Raise Hold

Set a timer and stand on tip toe for 60 seconds in total. Split into manageable sets.

Extra Credit: in one go, heels not touching the floor

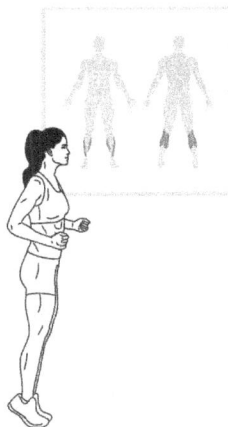

60

20 Forward Bends

Place your hands behind your head and bend forward. Repeat 20 times in total. Split into manageable sets.

Extra Credit: in one go

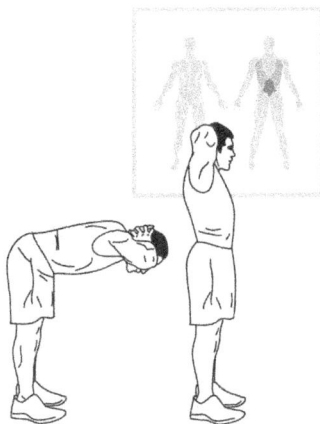

61

60 Seconds O-Pose Hold

Set a timer, sit down on the floor, lift your feet and arms up as illustrated and hold the pose for 60 seconds in total. Split into manageable sets.

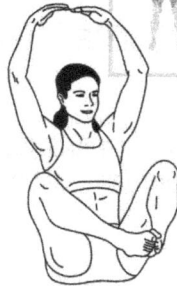

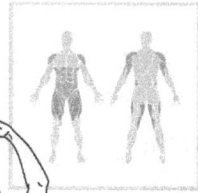

Extra Credit: in one go

62

60 Seconds Uneven Plank

Set a timer and hold an uneven plank for 30 seconds; switch sides and hold it for another 30 = 60 seconds in total. Split into manageable sets.

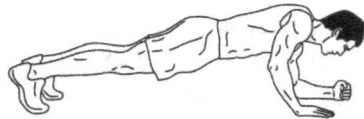

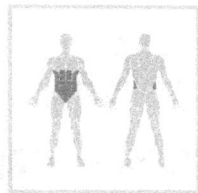

Extra Credit: in one go

30 Half Shrimp Squats

Stand on one leg and grab the other one as illustrated and do squats - 30 in total. Split into manageable sets.

Extra Credit: 15 / 15 in one go

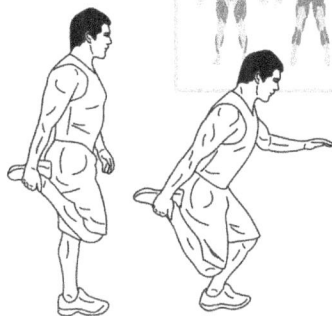

60 Seconds Half Jacks

Set a timer and do half jacks for 60 seconds in total. Split into manageable sets.

Extra Credit: non-stop

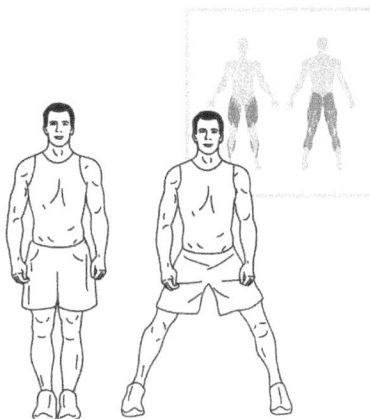

20 Raised Leg Circles

Get down on the floor and raise your legs at roughly 45 degrees. "Draw" circles in the air - 20 in total. Split into manageable sets.

Extra Credit: in one go

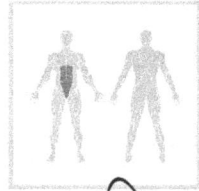

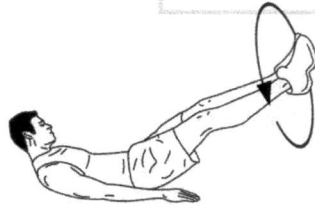

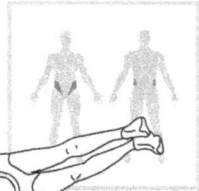

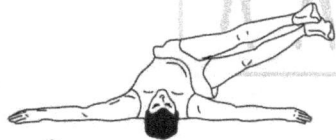

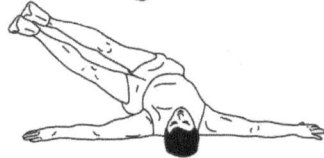

20 Windshield Wipers

Lie down on the floor or a bed, raise your legs up at 90 degrees. Tilt them to the left and then tilt them to the right (= 2 reps) 20 times in total (10 / 10 each side)

Extra Credit: in one go

67

40 Single-Leg Bridges

Lie down on the floor, raise one leg up as illustrated. Lift your torso up - 40 times in total; 20 times per side. Split into manageable sets.

Extra Credit: 20 / 20, in one go

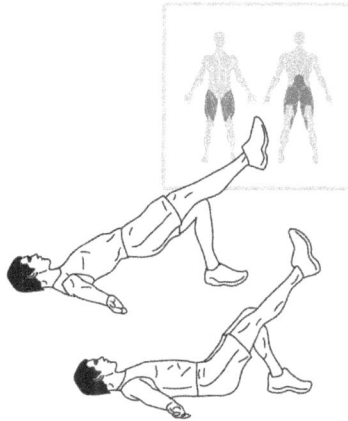

68

20 Crunch Kicks

Sit down on the floor as illustrated, raise your legs up at roughly 45 degrees and do crunch kicks - 20 in total. Split into manageable sets.

Extra Credit: in one go, don't lower your legs down

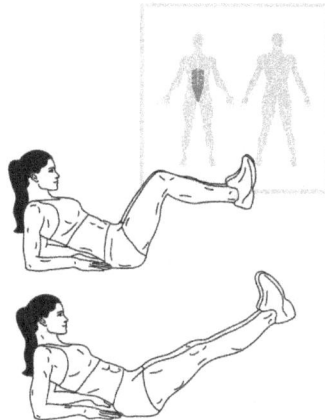

69

10 Cross Tricep Extensions

Get into a plank position, hands crossed over each other. Lower yourself down until your elbows touch the floor = 10 times in total. Split into manageable sets.

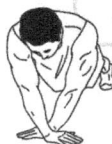

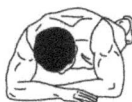

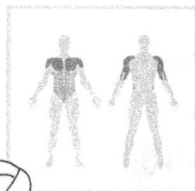

Extra Credit: in one go

70

80 Hooks

Throw hooks until you hit 80 reps in total. Split into manageable sets.

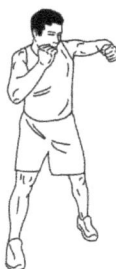

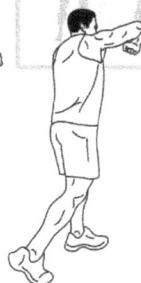

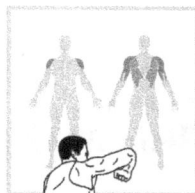

Extra Credit: in one go

40 Squat Hold Side Bends

Lower yourself into a squat and place your arms behind your head, as illustrated. Bend to the side and reach with your elbow to your knee - 40 times in total. Split into manageable sets.

Extra Credit: in one go

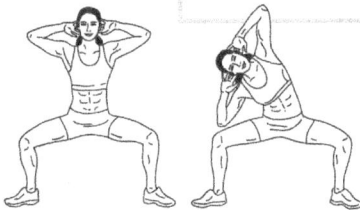

30 Seconds Star Plank

Get into a plank position, slide your arms and legs as far apart as you can and hold it for 30 seconds in total. Split into manageable sets.

Extra Credit: non-stop, keep the plank

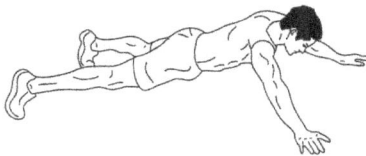

73

2 Minute Side Elbow Plank

Set a timer and hold a side plank for 1 minute; change sides and hold it for another minute = 2 minutes in total. Split into manageable sets.

Extra Credit: in one go

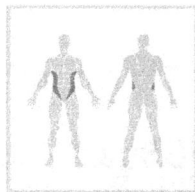

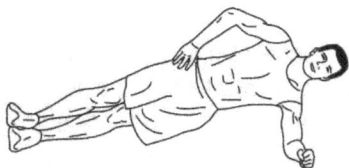

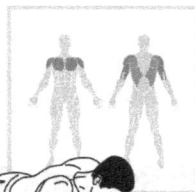

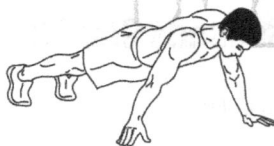

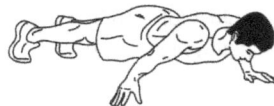

74

10 Archer Push-Ups

Get into a plank, one arm extended away from you and do 10 push-ups in total. Split into manageable sets. Switch sides with every rep.

Extra Credit: in one go

75

30 Seconds Raised Leg Hold

Set a timer, lie down and raise your legs at 45 degrees. Hold them up for 30 seconds in total.

Extra Credit: in one go

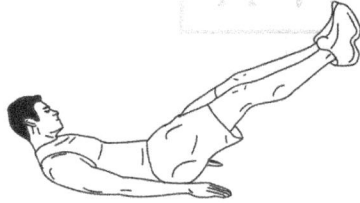

76

20 Reverse Plank Kicks

Get into a reverse plank, bring your knee in and push your foot away 20 times in total; 10 on the left eg, 10 on the right leg.

Extra Credit: 10 / 10 in one go

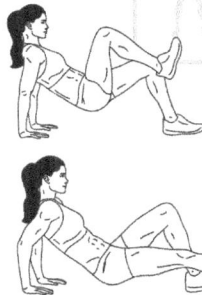

77

60 Seconds Chest Squeeze

Stand upright with both arms out in front of you, bent at a 90 degree angle. Lock your hands together and squeeze as hard as you can. Hold the contraction for 60 seconds in total.

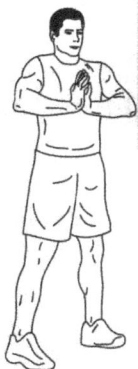

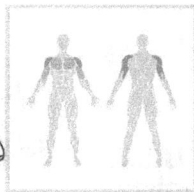

Extra Credit: non-stop

78

40 Front Kicks

Do front kicks until you hit 40 in total. Split into manageable sets.

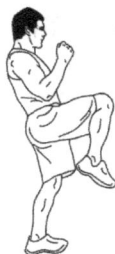

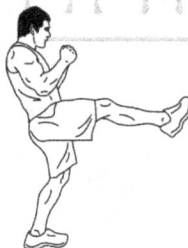

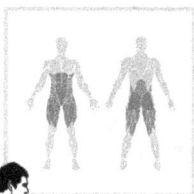

Extra Credit: 20/20, in one go
Extra Extra Credit: foot not touching the floor

79

10 V-Ups

Lie down on the floor and fold into a
V-Up, as illustrated, -10 times in total.
Split into manageable sets.

Extra Credit: in one go

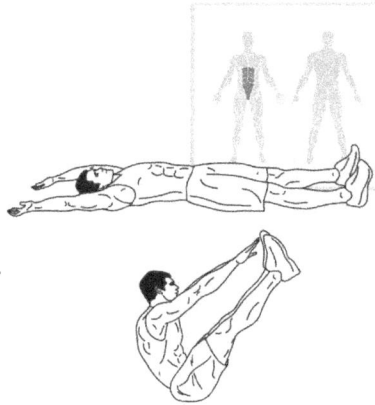

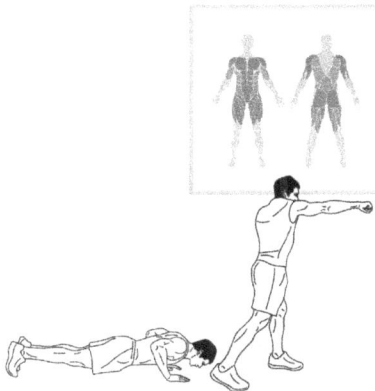

80

10 Push-Up + Jab + Cross

Drop into a push-up then jump up
and throw a jab followed up by a
cross. Repeat until you hit
10 in total. Split into manageable
sets.

Extra Credit: in one go

60 Side-to-Side Chops

"Chop" side to side, as illustrated, until you hit 60 chops in total. Split into manageable sets.

Extra Credit: in one go

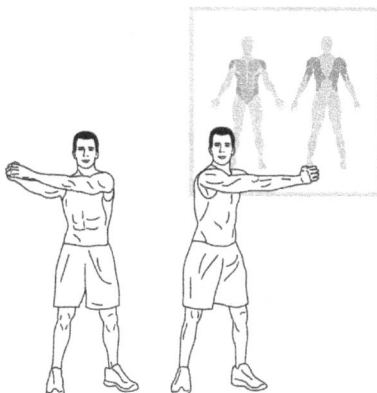

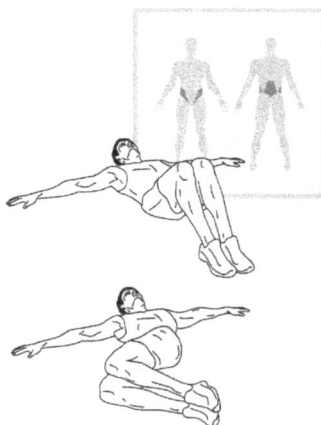

40 Knee Rolls

Lie down, knees bent as illustrated. Roll them from side to side, until they touch the floor - 40 times in total. Split into manageable sets.

Extra Credit: in one go

83

30 Get-Ups

Sit down on the floor, lean on one
arm and hold the other extended
above your shoulder. Liift yourself up
as illustrated - 30 times in total Split
into manageable sets.

Extra Credit: in one go

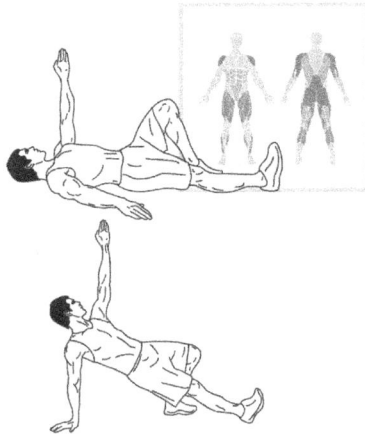

84

2 Minutes Single Leg
Hops on the Spot

Set a timer and hop on one leg for 2
minutes in total; 60 seconds per leg.
Split into manageable sets.

Extra Credit: non-stop

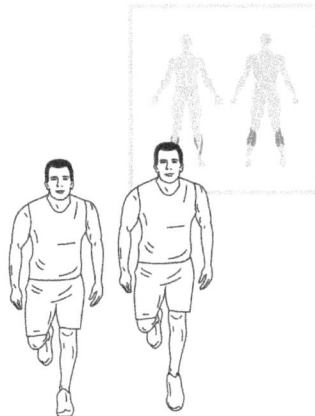

85

30 Side Plank Rotations

Get into a side elbow plank, slide your hand under your torso and bring it up towards the ceiling as illustrated. 15 left side, 15 right side = 30 times in total. Split into manageable sets.

Extra Credit: in one go

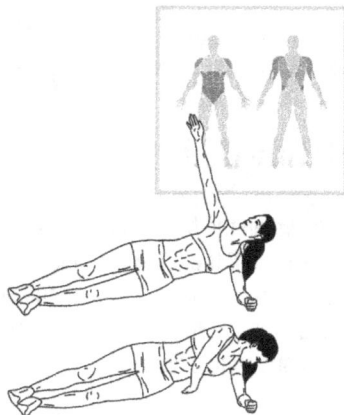

86

30 Split Lunges

Step into a lunge and go up, without moving off the spot, as illustrated. Repeat 30 times in total - 15 left side, 15 right side. Split into manageable sets.

Extra Credit: 15/15 in one go

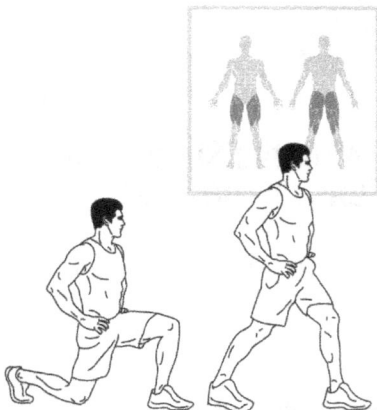

87

15 Basic Burpees With a Jump

Do basic burpees with a jump (no push-up) as fast as you can until you hit 15 in total. Split into manageable sets.

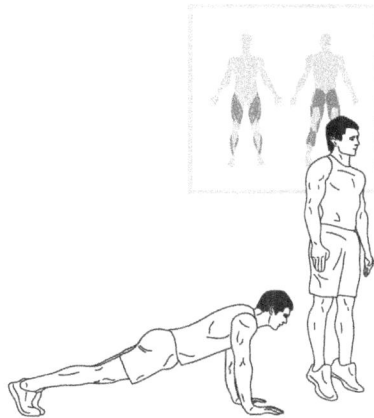

Extra Credit: in one go

88

200 Overhead Punches

Do overhead punches, 100 with the right arm, 100 with the left arm, 200 times in total. Complete one side first before starting on the other. Split into manageable sets.

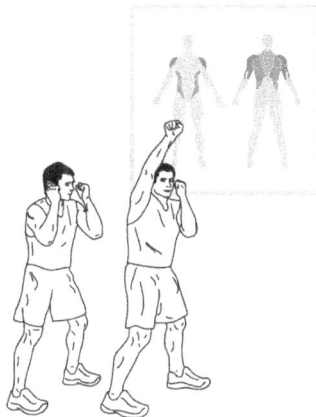

Extra Credit: 150/150, in one go

89

30 Thigh Taps

Get into a plank position and tap your
thighs - 30 times in total.
Split into manageable sets.

Extra Credit: in one go

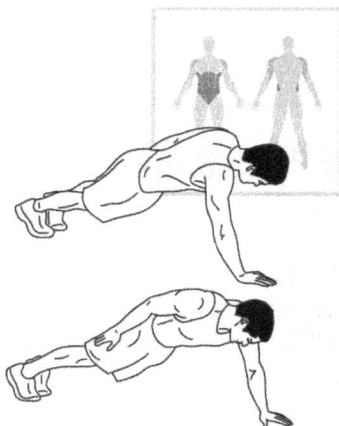

90

60 Seconds Tree Pose

Hold the Tree Pose (as illustrated) for
30 seconds in one go, change sides
and hold it for another 30 seconds.

Extra Credit: in one go, keep balance

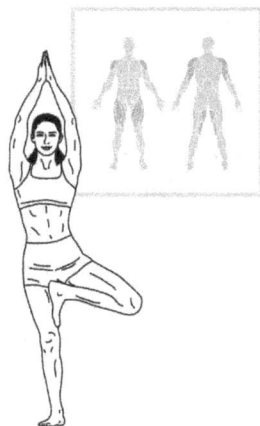

91

30 Squat Hops
on the Spot

Place your hands behind your head
and lower yourself into a deep squat.
Hop on the spot, without getting up,
30 times in total. Split into manageable sets.

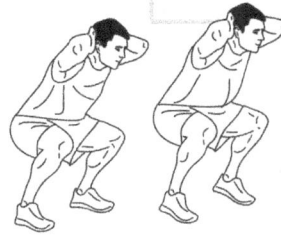

Extra Credit: in one go

92

60 Seconds Reverse
Plank Hold

Get into a reverse plank position
as illustrated - and hold it for 60
seconds in total.
Split into manageable sets.

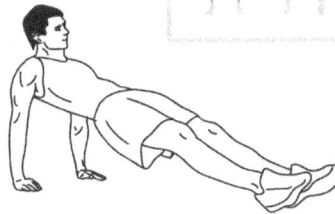

Extra Credit: in one go

93

40 Knee-to-Elbow Crunches

Get on the floor, place your hands behind your head and bring the opposite knee to opposite elbow 40 times in total.

Extra Credit: in one go

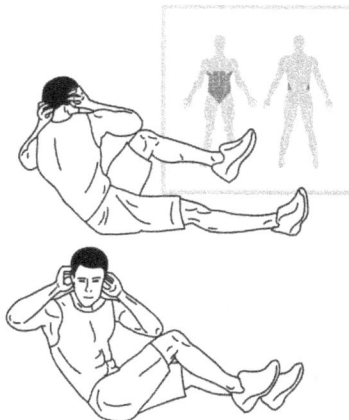

94

40 Half Shrimp Squats

Stand on one leg and grab the other one as illustrated and do squats - 40 in total. Split into manageable sets.

Extra Credit: 20 / 20, in one go

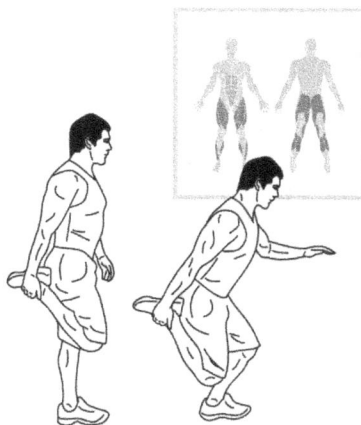

40 Side Bridges

Get into a side elbow plank, lower
your hips to the floor and come up
again - 40 times in total; 20 per side.
Split into manageable sets.

Extra Credit: 20/ 20 in one go

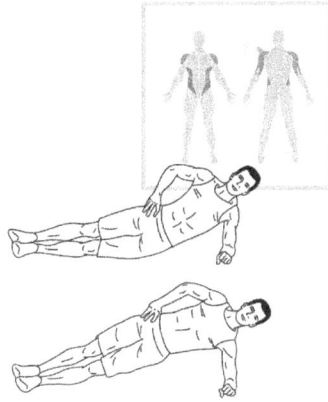

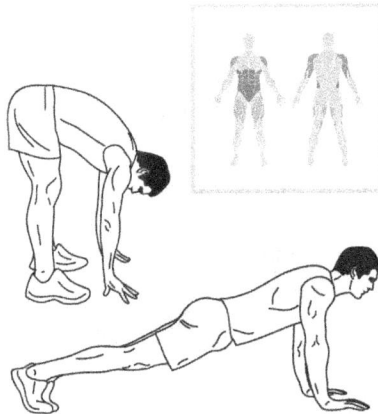

15 Plank Walk-Outs

Walk out into a plank, as illustrated,
until you hit 15 in total. Split into
manageable sets.

Extra Credit: in one go

30 Sit-Ups

Lie down on the floor and do sit-ups until you hit 30 in total. Split into manageable sets.

Extra Credit: in one go

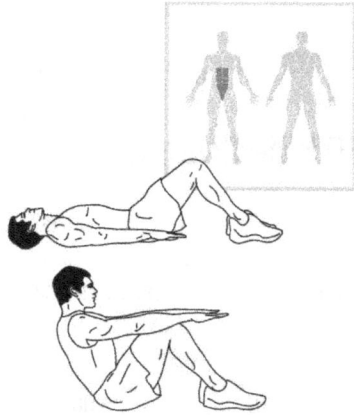

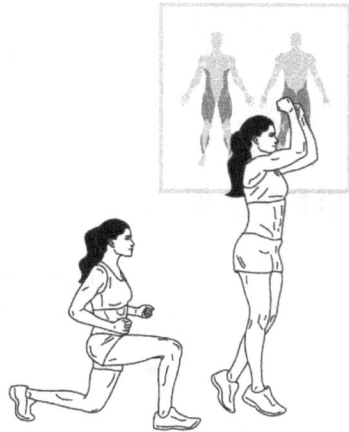

20 Jumping Lunges

Jump up and land into a lunge, try to jump as high as you can each time. Complete 10 reps on one side, then 10 reps on the other side = 20 times in total. Split into manageable sets.

Extra Credit: in one go

99

30 Seconds Tricep Dip Hold

Lower yourself into a tricep dip and hold it for 30 seconds in total. Split into manageable sets.

Extra Credit: in one go

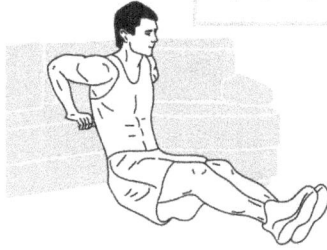

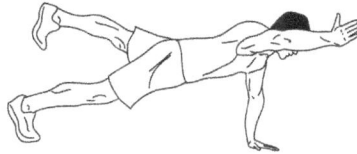

100

2 Minutes Alt Arm/Leg Raised Plank

Set a timer and get into a plank position. Raise your left arm and your right leg up and hold it for 2 minutes in total. Change arm/leg halfway through (60 seconds per side). Split into manageable sets.

Extra Credit: in one go

101

10 Diamond Push-Ups

Get into a plank position, bring your hands together forming a "diamond" and do push-ups - 10 in total. Split into manageable sets.

Extra Credit: in one go

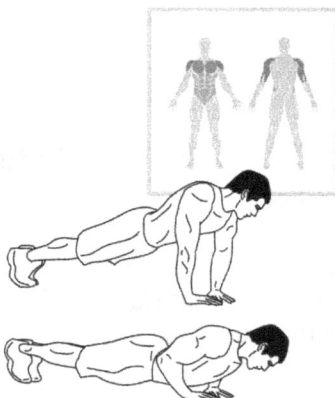

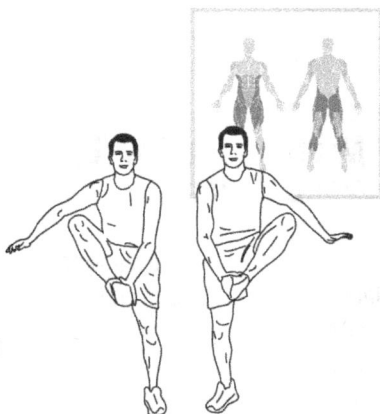

102

60 Seconds Toe Tap Hops

Set a timer, hop up and tap your opposite toe with the opposite hand, as fast as you can, for 60 seconds in total. Split into manageable sets.

Extra Credit: in one go

103

60 Shoulder Taps

Get into a plank position and tap your left shoulder - 30 times, then tap your right houlder 30 times; 60 times in total.

Extra Credit: in one go, keep the plank

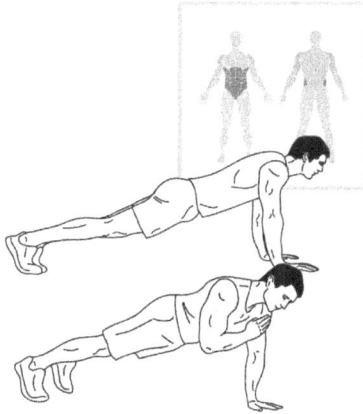

104

20 Single Leg Deadlifts

Start standing on left leg with right leg lifted and bent at a 90-degree angle in front of body. Bend forward, hands reaching toward the floor as right leg extends directly behind the body. Repeat 20 times in total, 10 per side.

Extra Credit: 10/10, in one go

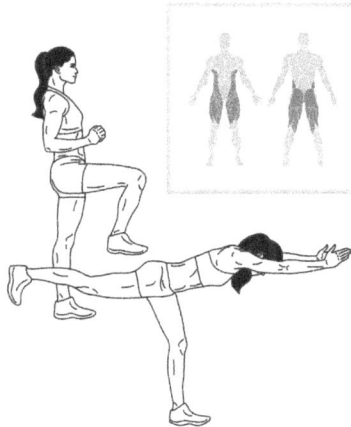

105

30 Dead Bugs

Lay down on the floor with your
hands extended above you toward
the ceiling. Bend your knees in 90
degree angle. Slowly lower the
opposite arm and the opposite leg
down to the floor simultaneously.
Repeat 30 times in total.

Extra Credit: in one go

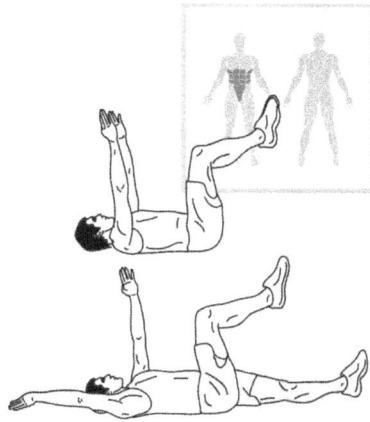

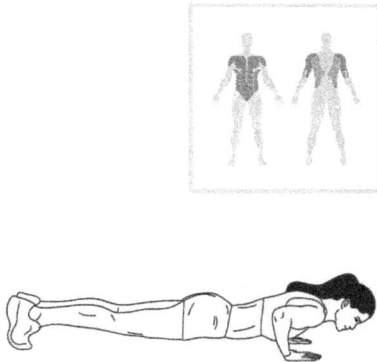

106

20 Seconds Push-Up
Plank Hold

Get into a plank and lower yourself
down into a push-up - hold it for
20 seconds in total.

Extra Credit: in one go

107

5 Pop-Ups

Kneel on the floor, sitting back on heels. Raise arms overhead, then throw arms back behind body before driving them forward and explosively popping up off knees to land on feet. Perform a tuck jump - 5 times in total.

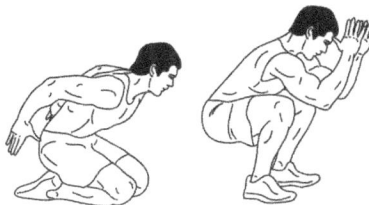

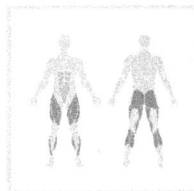

Extra Credit: in one go

108

30 Seconds Plank Leg Raises

Set a timer and do plank leg raises for 30 seconds in total;
Split into manageable sets. Change legs halfway through.

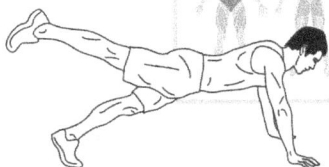

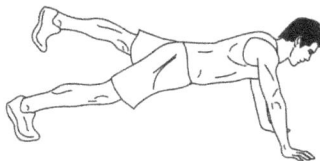

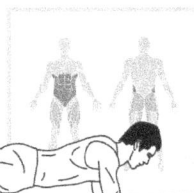

Extra Credit: in one go

109

30 Seconds Pacer Steps

Set a timer and lower yourself into a squat. Pace on the spot while in a squat position as fast as you can - 30 seconds in total.

Extra Credit: in one go

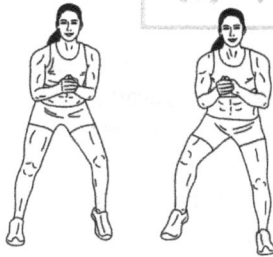

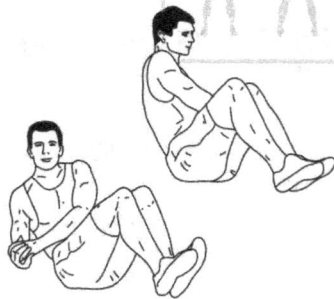

110

30 Sitting Twists

Sit down on the floor or a sofa and do sitting twists, as illustrated - 30 in total. Split into manageable sets.

Extra Credit: in one go

30 Push-Ups

Get into a plank position and do a push-up until you hit 30 in total. Split into manageable sets.

Extra Credit: in one go

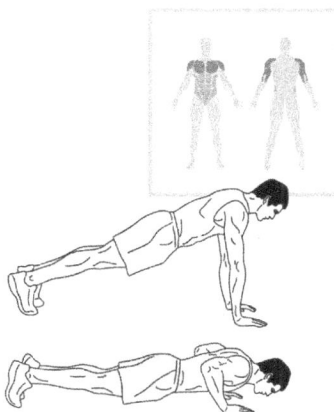

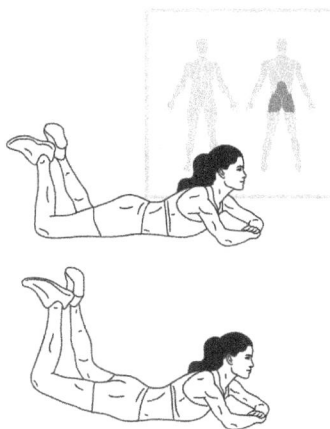

20 Glute Flex

Lie down on your stomach, legs bent at 90 degrees, heels together. Raise your buttocks off the flor as high as you can - 20 times in total.

Extra Credit: in one go

113

80 Climbers

Get down into a plank. Begin to climb
on the spot, as fast as you can, until
you hit 80 reps in total (40 per leg).
Split into manageable sets.

Extra Credit: in one go

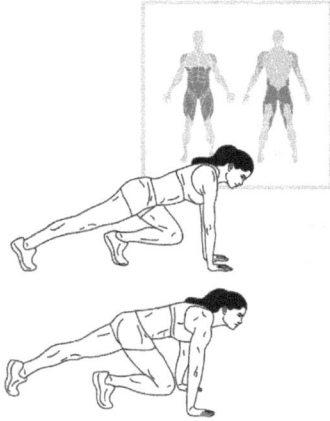

114

2 Minutes Plank
Punches

Set a timer and get into a plank.
Throw punches as fast as you can
for 2 minutes in total. Split into
manageable sets.

Extra Credit: non-stop

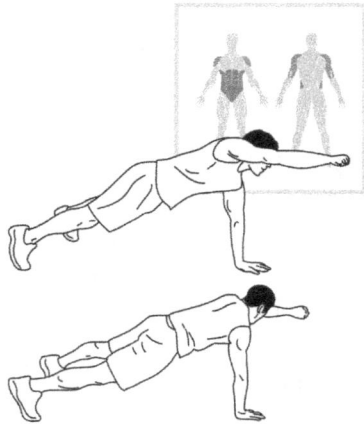

115

80 Standing Shoulder Taps

Tap your shoulders and raise your arms up reaching for the ceiling - 80 times in total. Split into manageable sets.

Extra Credit: in one go

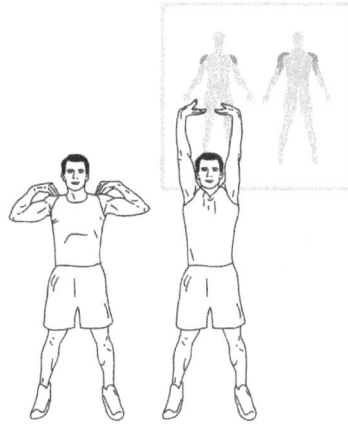

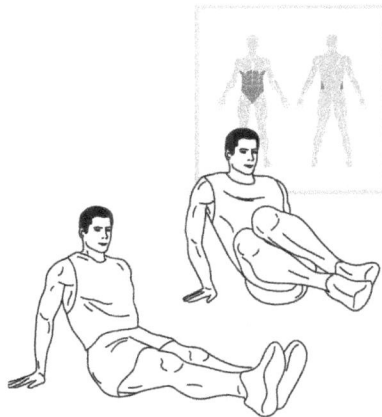

116

50 Knee In & Twists

Sit down on the floor, legs extended in front of you. Bring your knees in while twisting them to your side. Repeat 50 times in total. Split into manageable sets.

Extra Credit: in one go

80 Side Leg Raises

Raise your right leg to your side
at 90 degrees until you hit 40 reps;
change legs and do another 40,
60 in total. You can hold on to
something.

Extra Credit: 40/40 in one go

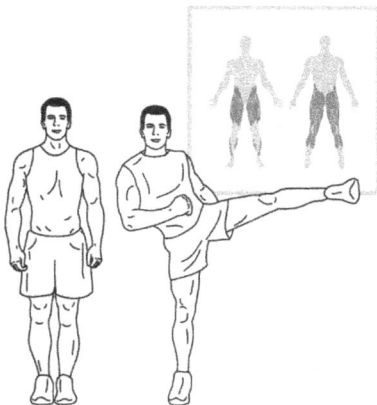

2 Minutes Butt Kicks

Set a timer and do butt kicks for
2 minutes in total. Split into manageable sets.

Extra Credit: non-stop

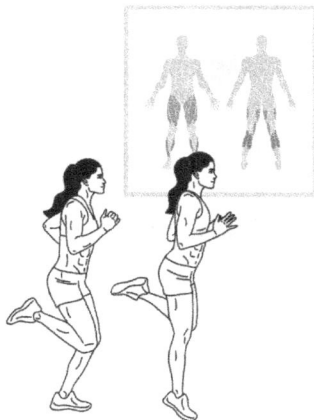

60 Seconds Palm Strikes

Set a timer and do palm strikes for 60 seconds in total. Split into manageable sets.

Extra Credit: in one go

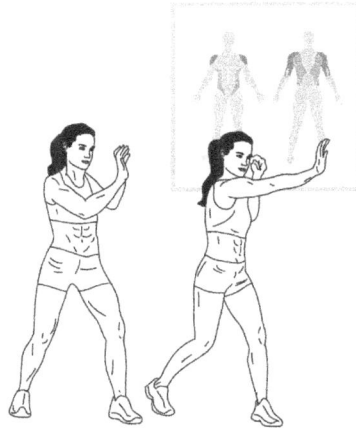

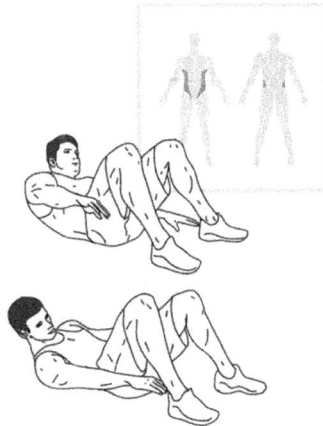

40 Heel Taps

Lie down on the floor as illustrated, reach for, and then tap your heels - 40 times in total. Split into manageable sets.

Extra Credit: in one go

121

20 Side V-Ups

Lie down on your side, legs extended straight, one arm behind your head. Fold your body up (into a V) so your elbow touches your knee - 20 times in total. Split into manageable sets.

Extra Credit: 10/10, in one go

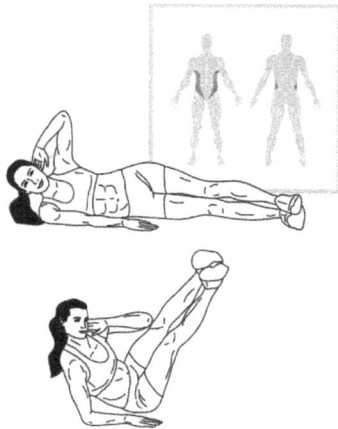

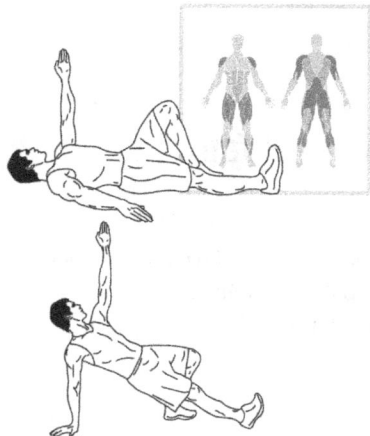

122

40 Get-Ups

Sit down on the floor, lean on one arm and hold the other extended above your shoulder. Liift yourself up as illustrated - 40 times in total. Split into manageable sets.

Extra Credit: in one go

60 Leg Extensions

Get on your hands and knees and raise your left leg up bent at 90 degrees - continue until you hit 30 repetitions in total; switch legs halfway and do another 30. Split into manageable sets.

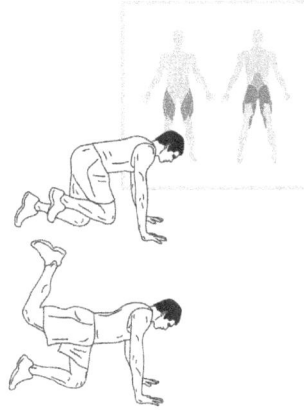

Extra Credit: 30/30, in one go

40 Balance Back Kicks

Balance on one leg and kick back with the other as illustrated - 40 times in total; 20 per leg.

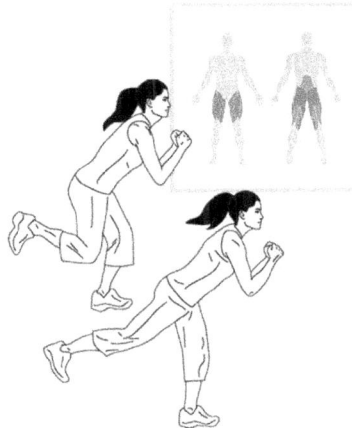

Extra Credit: 20/20, in one go

125

60 Squats

Do squats until you hit 60 in total.
Split into manageabe sets - as fewer
as possible.

Extra Credit: in one go

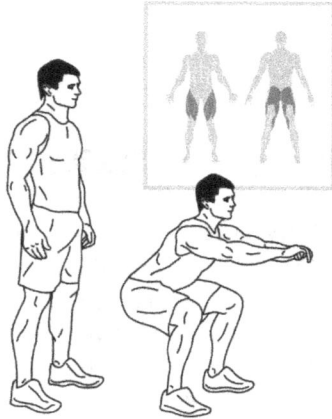

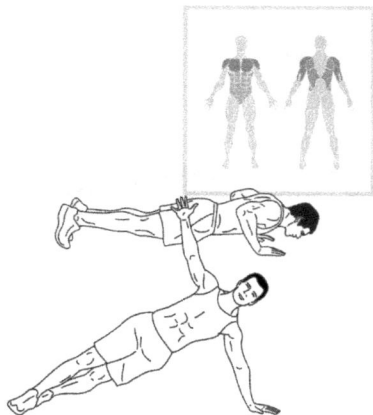

126

20 Push-Up
With Rotations

Get on the floor and lower yourself
into a push-up, come up and turn
into a side plank - 20 times in total;
split into manageable sets.

Extra Credit: in one go

127

60 Seconds High Knees

Set a timer and do high knees (sprint on the spot) for 60 seconds in total. Split into manageable sets.

Extra Credit: non-stop

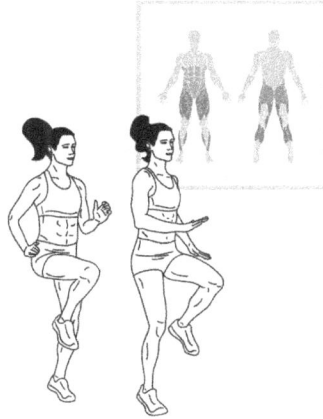

128

60 Calf Raises

Stand up straight, arms behind your back and raise up onto your toes - 60 times in total. Split into manageable sets.

Extra Credit: in one go

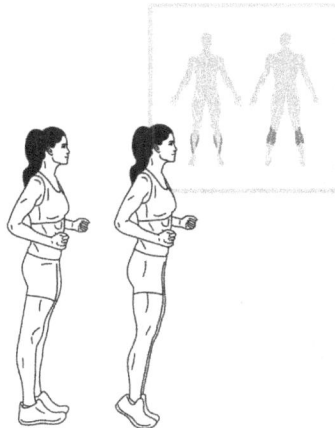

129

20 Scapula Shrugs

Get into a plank position and squeeze your shoulder blades together - it will lower your torso slightly. Do not bend your arms. Repeat 20 times in total.

Extra Credit: in one go

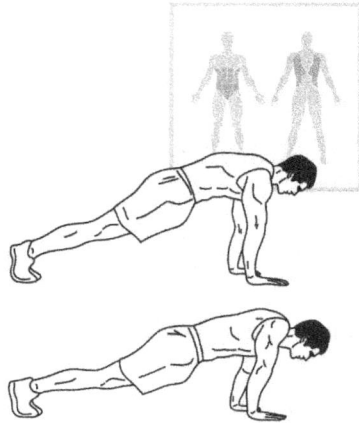

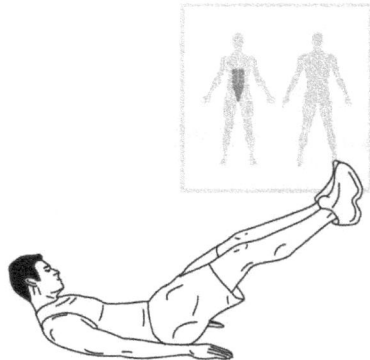

130

60 Seconds Raised Leg Hold

Set a timer, lie down and raise your legs at 45 degrees. Hold them up for 60 seconds in total.

Extra Credit: in one go

131

30 Bridge Taps

Lie down, raise your hips up and tap the floor over your head. Repeat 30 times in total. Split into manageable sets.

Extra Credit: in one go

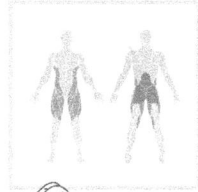

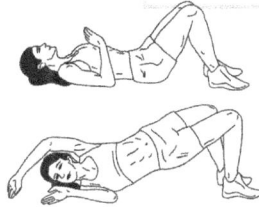

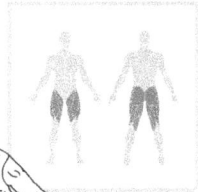

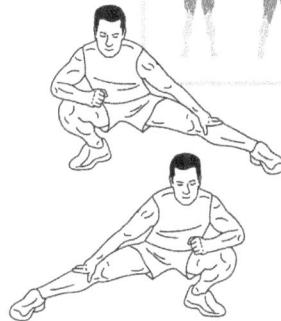

132

50 Side-To-Side Lunges

Get into a deep side lunge position and shift your body to the other side without standing up, 50 times in total. Split into manageable sets.

Extra Credit: in one go

133

40 Squat + Step Back

Lower yourself into a deep squat and place your hands on your knees so your elbows point to your sides as illustrated, then step back - 40 times in total. Split into manageable sets.

Extra Credit: in one go

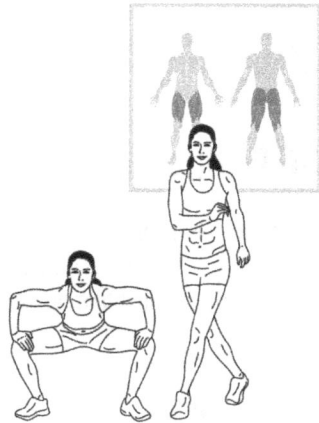

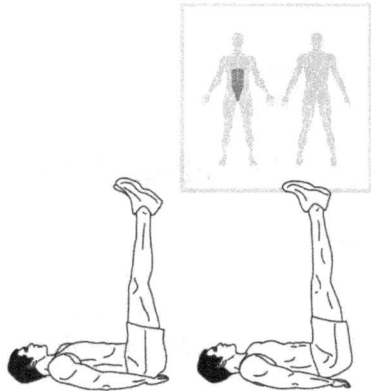

134

30 Pulse Ups

Lie down, raise your legs up at a 90 degrees angle and lift your hips off the floor slightly. Pulse up and down as illustrated 30 times in total.

Extra Credit: in one go

50 Side Bridges

Get into a side elbow plank, lower
your hips to the floor and come up
again - 50 times in total; 25 per side.
Split into manageable sets.

Extra Credit: 25/25 in one go

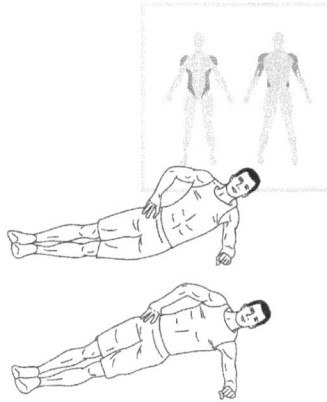

60 Seconds Half Bow

Set a timer and raise your arms fingers pointing up. Bend your elbows
so your fingers point forward, as
illustrated - for 60 seconds in total.
Split into manageable sets.

Extra Credit: non-stop

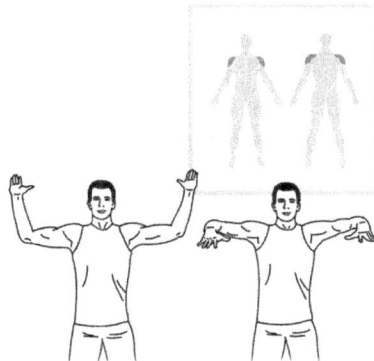

137

60 Seal Jacks

Start with your arms raised to
your sides, legs wide then jump in,
bringing your hands together.
Repeat 60 times in total.

Extra Credit: in one go

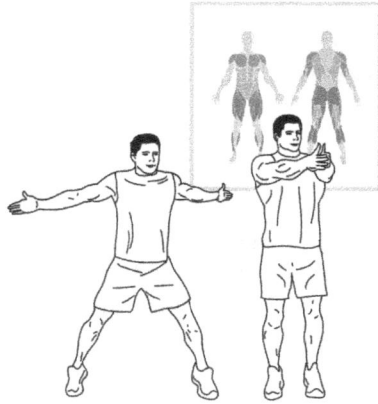

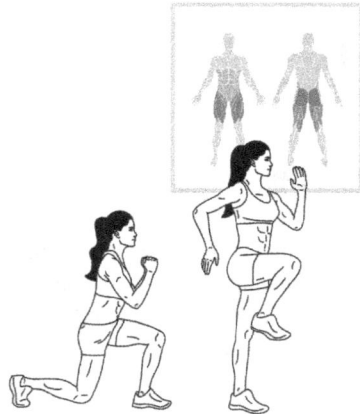

138

50 Lunge Step-Ups

Start from a lunge and step up 50
times in total, 25 times per side
(complete one side first, then the
other). Split into manageable sets.

Extra Credit: in one go

139

30 Push-Up With Rotations

Get on the floor and lower yourself into a push-up, come up and turn into a side plank - 30 times in total; split into manageable sets.

Extra Credit: in one go

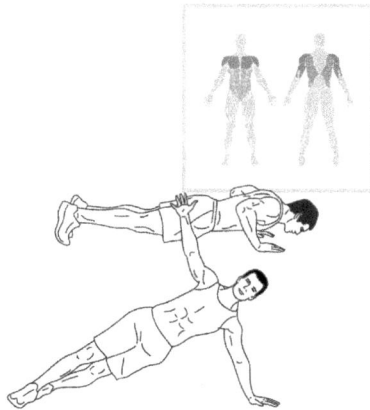

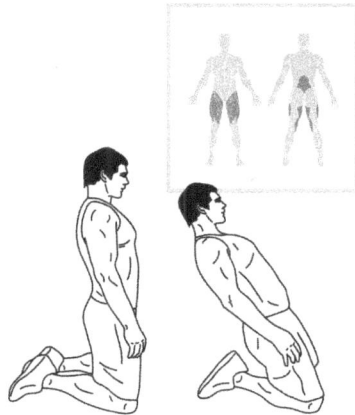

140

15 Matrix Tilts

Kneel, body upright, thighs straight. Slowly lean back at roughly 15 degree angle and then slowly return to starting position. That's one rep. Repeat 20 times in total.

Extra Credit: in one go

141

2 Minutes March Steps

Set a timer and do march steps
(march on the spot) for 2 minutes in
total. Split into manageable sets.

Extra Credit: non-stop

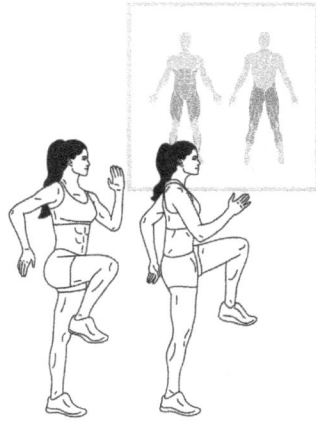

142

30 Infinity Circles

Raise your leg to the side, waist
height and draw infinity symbol in
the air - 30 in total, 15 each leg. Split
into manageable sets.

Extra Credit: in one go

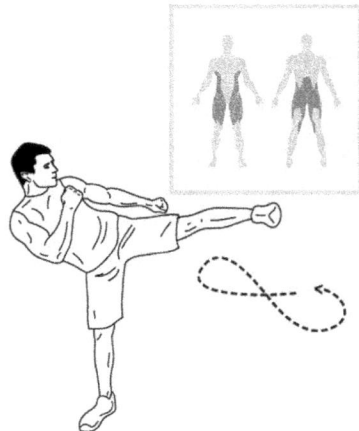

143

2 Minutes Uneven Plank

Set a timer and hold an uneven plank for 60 seconds; switch sides and hold it for another 60 = 2 minutes in total. Split into manageable sets.

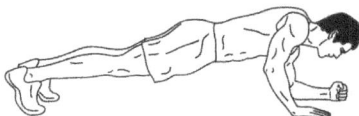

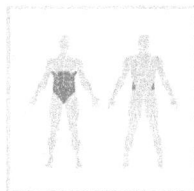

Extra Credit: in one go

144

10 Jump Knee Tucks

Jump up bringing your knees to your chest - 10 times in total.
Split into manageable sets.

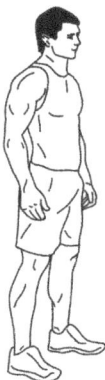

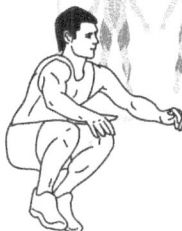

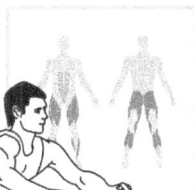

Extra Credit: in one go

100 Standing Shoulder Taps

Tap your shoulders and raise your arms up reaching for the ceiling - 100 times in total. Split into manageable sets.

Extra Credit: in one go

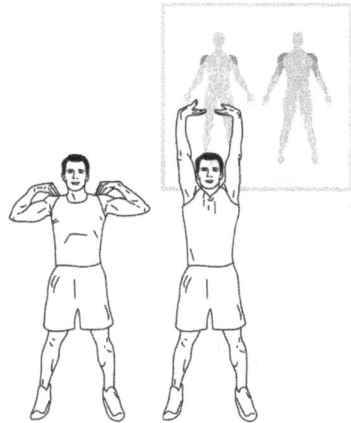

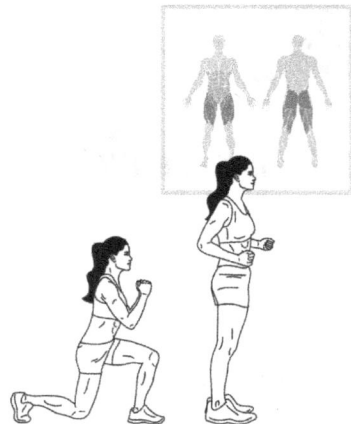

40 Reverse Lunges

Step back into a lunge - 40 times in total. Split into manageable sets.

Extra Credit: in one go

147

30 Butterfly Dips

Sit down on the floor and lean back, heels together. Lift yourself up bringing your knees together. Repeat 30 times in total. Split into manageable sets.

Extra Credit: in one go

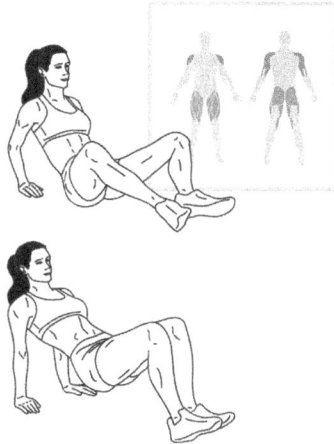

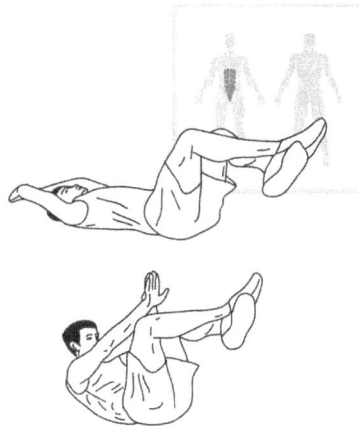

148

50 Knee Crunches

Lie down on the floor, bring your knees up and lean forward until your elbows and knees touch - 50 times in total. Split into manageable sets.

Extra Credit: in one go

149

30 Plank Rotations

Get into a plank and do rotations as illustrated until you hit 30 in total. Split into manageable sets.

Extra Credit: in one go

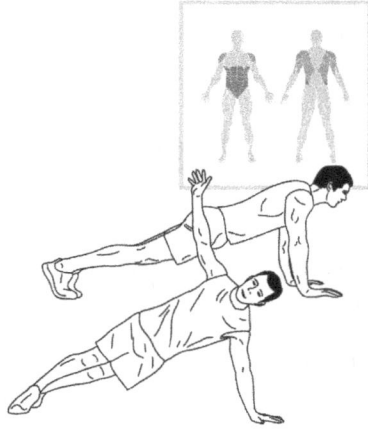

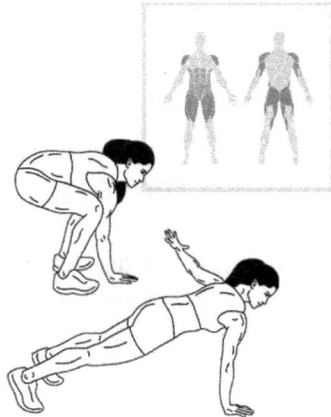

150

10 Single Arm Plank Jump-Ins

Get into a one-armed plank position - jump in and then back out 10 times in total (5 each arm); Split into manageable sets.

Extra Credit: in one go

151

30 Lunges With Twist

Raise your arms in front of you and step forward into a lunge, twisting your body to the side. Repeat 30 times in total. Split into manageable sets.

Extra Credit: 15/15, in one go

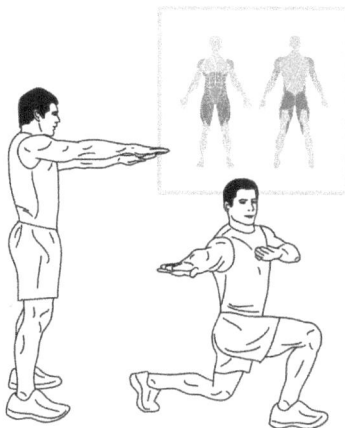

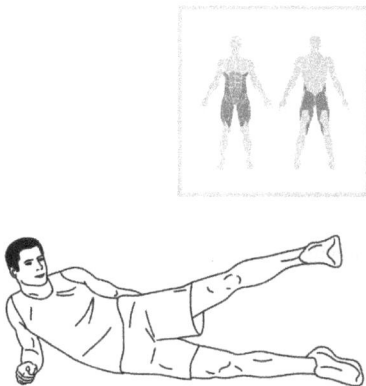

152

2 Minutes Leg Raise Hold

Lie down on the floor on your side and raise your leg at about 30 degrees - as illustrated. Hold it up for 2 minutes in total, 60 seconds per side. Split into manageable sets.

Extra Credit: in one go

153

60 Seconds Turning Kicks

Set a timer and do turning kicks for 60 seconds in total. Switch sides halfway through.

Extra Credit: in one go

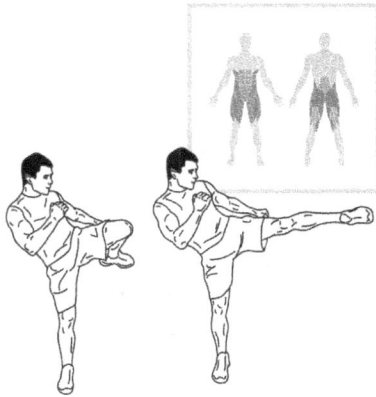

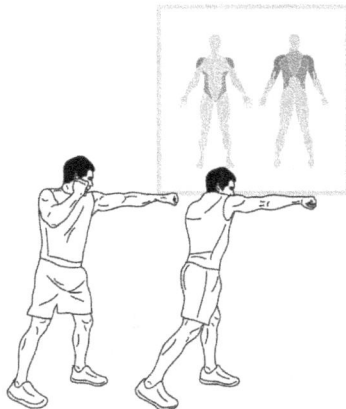

154

5 Minutes Punches

Set a timer and punch (jab + cross) for 5 minutes in total. Split into manageable sets.

Extra Credit: in one go

155

20 Superman Extensions

Lie down on the floor, stretch your arms in front of you and do superman extensions as illustrated. Split into manageable sets.

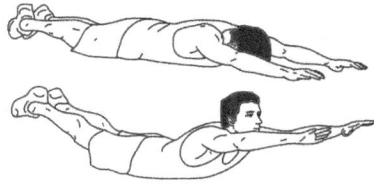

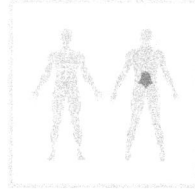

Extra Credit: in one go

156

4 Minute Side Elbow Plank

Set a timer and hold a side plank for 2 minutes; change sides and hold it for another 2 minutes = 4 minutes in total. Split into manageable sets.

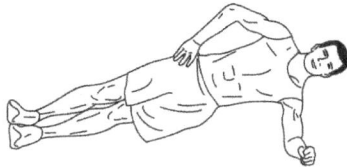

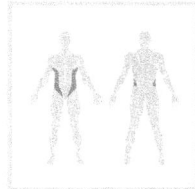

Extra Credit: in one go

157

5 Reverse Grip Push-Ups

Get into a plank position and reverse your grip with your fingers pointing towards your toes. Perform 5 push-ups in total. Split into manageable sets.

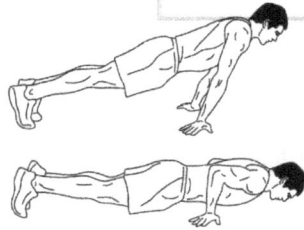

Extra Credit: in one go

158

40 Balance Side Lunges

Raise your arms and one knee up. Step to the side into a lunge - 40 times in total. Split into manageable sets.

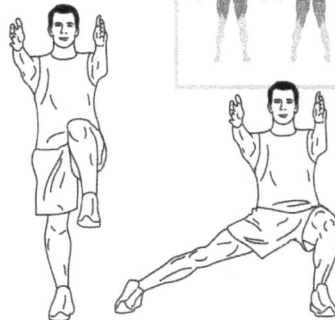

Extra Credit: in one go,

keep arms up

159

5 Minutes Raised Arm Hold

Raise your arms to your sides at shoulder height and hold them up for 5 minutes in total. Split into manageable sets.

Extra Credit: in one go,
keep arms up

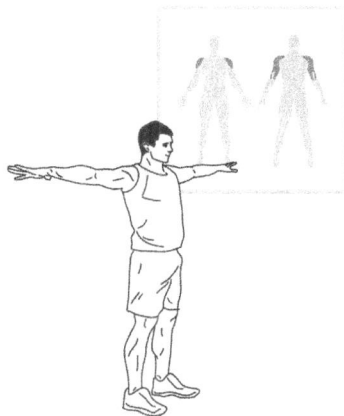

160

40 Squat Step-Ups

Squat and step up, as illustrated until you hit 20 reps, change sides and do another 20; 40 in total. Split into manageable sets.

Extra Credit: in one go

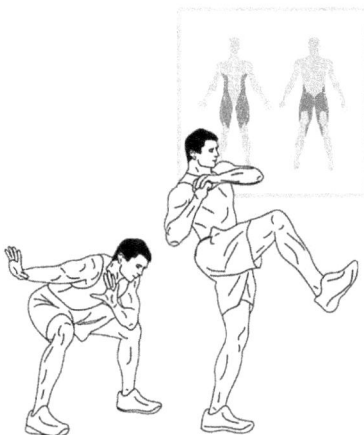

161

40 Reverse Plank Leg Raises

Get into a reverse plank as illustrated and raise your legs up - 40 times in total. Split into manageable sets.

Extra Credit: in one go

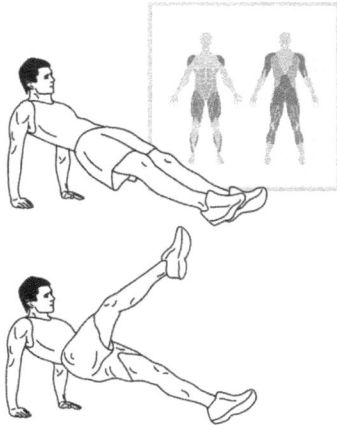

162

30 Raised Leg Crunches

Lie down and raise your legs off the floor. Keep your legs up and do crunches until you hit 30 in total. Split into manageable sets.

Extra Credit: in one go , keep legs up

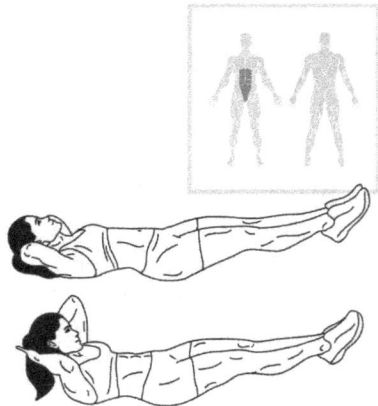

163

30 Full Bridges

Sit down on the floor as illustrated and raise your hips up as high as you can - 30 times in total. Split into manageable sets.

Extra Credit: in one go

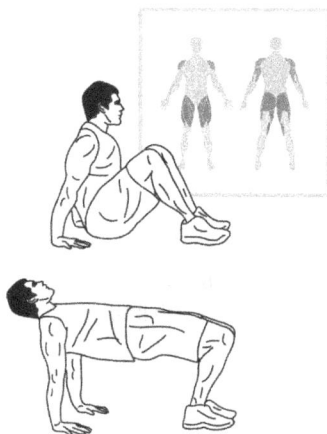

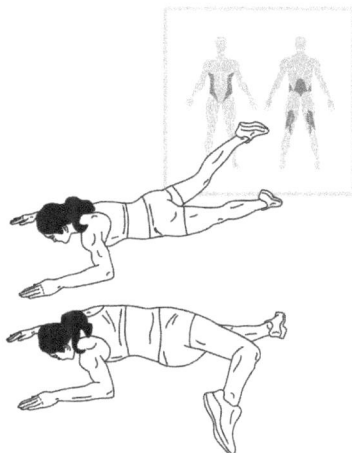

164

30 Scorpion Twists

Lie down on the floor, bend your right knee, and lift your right leg as high as you can then twist your hips and reach your right foot over to touch the ground on the outside of your left leg - 30 times in total; 15 times per side.

Extra Credit: in one go

30 Butt-Ups

Lie down on the floor, knees in.
Extend your legs towards the ceiling.
Repeat 30 times in total. Split into
manageable sets.

Extra Credit: in one go

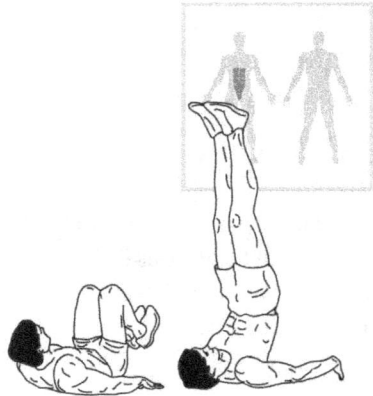

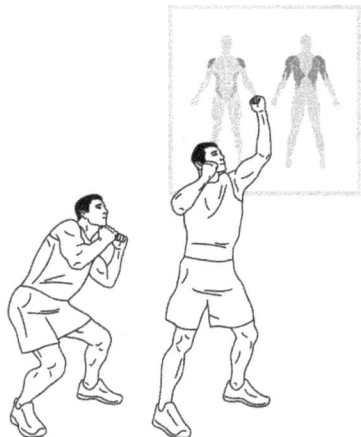

100 Uppercuts

Throw uppercuts until you hit 50.
Switch sides and throw another 50;
100 uppercuts in total . Split into
manageable sets.

Extra Credit: in one go

167

60 Seconds Squat Hold

Lower yourself into a squat (your glutes should be parallel to the floor) and hold it for 60 seconds in total. Split into manageable sets.

Extra Credit: in one go

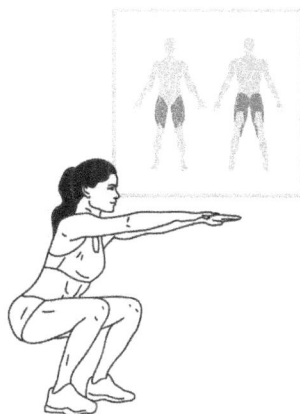

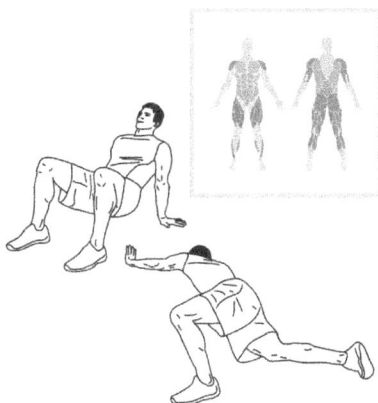

168

20 Swipers

Get on the floor into a relaxed table position and do swipers, as illustrated, 20 times in total. Split into manageable sets.

Extra Credit: in one go

70 Calf Raises

Stand up straight, arms behind your back and raise up onto your toes - 70 times in total. Split into manageable sets.

Extra Credit: in one go

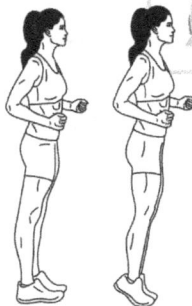

2 Minutes Elbow Clicks

Stand up straight with your arms raised shoulder height, elbows bent at 90 degrees. Bring your elbows together in front of you. Repeat as fast as you can for 2 minutes in total.

Extra Credit: non-stop

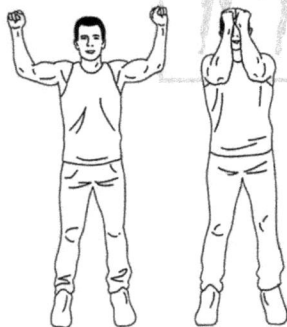

30 Air Circles

Raise your leg to the side, waist height and draw small circles n the air - 30 in total, 15 each leg. Sp it into manageable sets.

Extra Credit: in one go

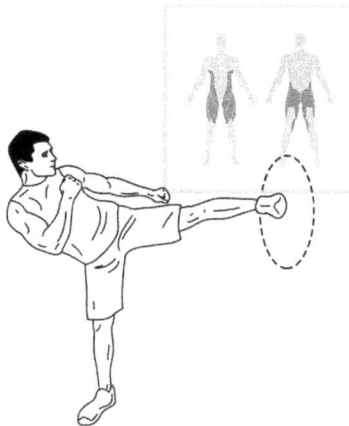

40 Cross Reach Sit-Ups

Lie down on the floor and raise one arm towards the ceiling. Sit-up and reach with opposite arm towards opposite foot- 40 times in total. Split into manageable sets.

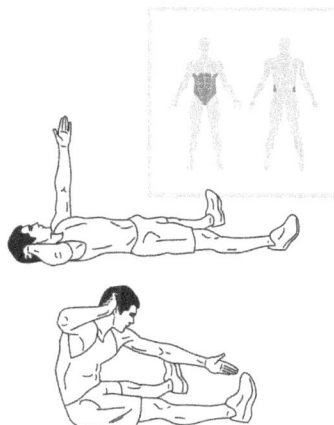

Extra Credit: in one go

30 Around The World

Crouch down and tap the floor behind you then lean forward and tap the floor in front of you. Repeat 30 times in total, 15 taps per side. Split into manageable sets.

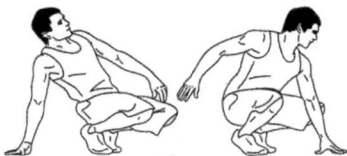

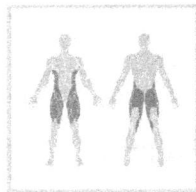

Extra Credit: in one go

30 Side Plank Knee Taps

Get into a side plank and tap your knee 15 times. Change sides and do another 15 taps, 30 taps in total. Split into manageable sets.

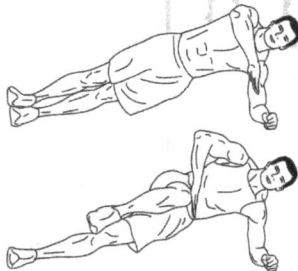

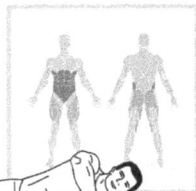

Extra Credit: in one go

175

30 Folded Crunches

Lie down on the floor and fold your legs to the side as illustrated. Do crunches - 30 in total, 15 per side. Split into manageable sets.

Extra Credit: in one go

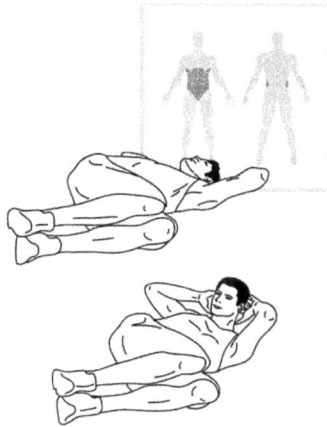

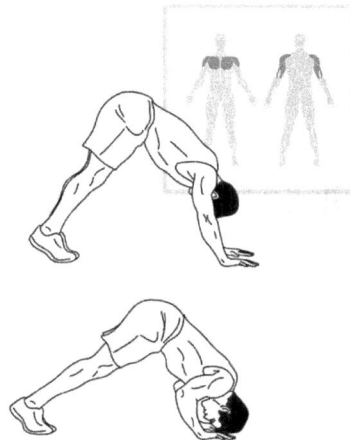

176

20 Pike Push-Ups

Get into a push-up position and lift up your hips so that your body forms an upside down V. Bend your elbows and lower your upper body until the top of your head nearly touches the floor - 20 times in total. Split into manageable sets.

Extra Credit: in one go

2 Minutes Side Splits

Set a timer and hold side splits (go as low as you can) for 2 minutes in total. Split into manageable sets.

Extra Credit: in one go

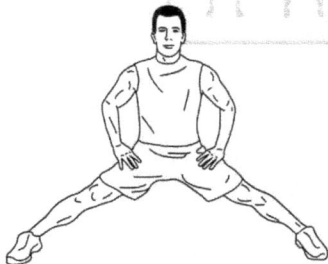

100 Knife Hand Strikes

Throw knife hand strikes until you hit 50. Change sides and throw another 50, 100 in total. Split into manageable sets.

Extra Credit: 50/50, in one go

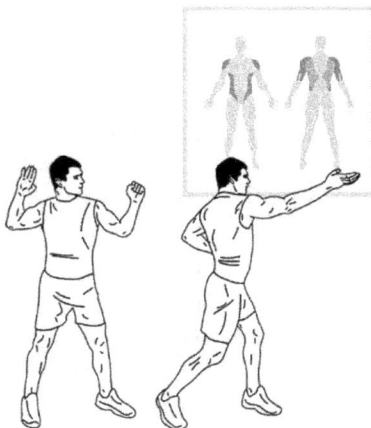

60 Hooks Kicks

Do hook kicks until you hit 60 in total; 30 per side. Split into manageable sets.

Extra Credit: 30/30, in one go
Extra Extra Credit: 30 in one go with foot not touching the floor

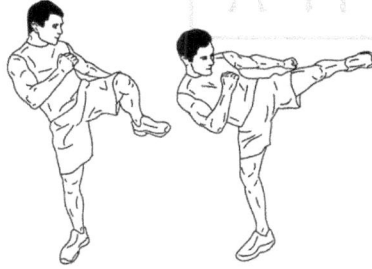

30 Modified Scissors

Lie down and raise your legs off the floor as illustrated. Move your legs apart and bring them back together - 30 times in total. Split into manageable sets.

Extra Credit: in one go

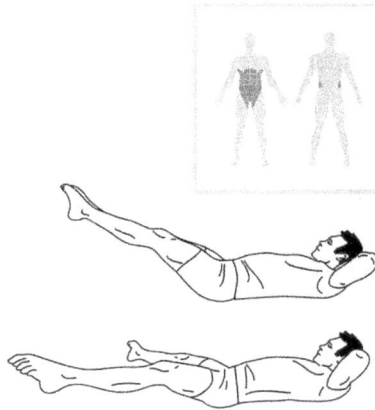

60 Knee In & Twists

Sit down on the floor, legs extended in front of you. Bring your knees in while twisting them to your side. Repeat 60 times in total. Split into manageable sets.

Extra Credit: in one go

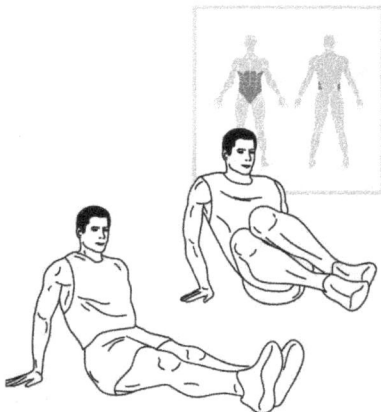

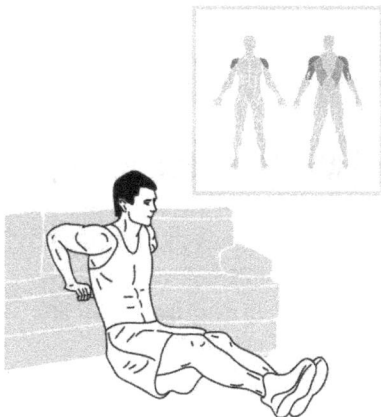

60 Seconds Tricep Dip Hold

Lower yourself into a tricep dip and hold it for 60 seconds in total. Split into manageable sets.

Extra Credit: in one go

2 Minutes High Knees

Set a timer and do high knees (sprint on the spot) for 2 minutes in total. Split into manageable sets.

Extra Credit: non-stop

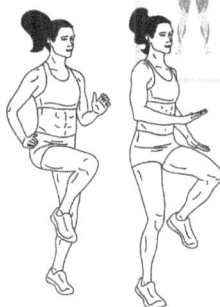

60 March Twists

March on the spot while twisting so your opposite elbow touches your opposite knee, as illustrated - 60 times in total.

Extra Credit: in one go

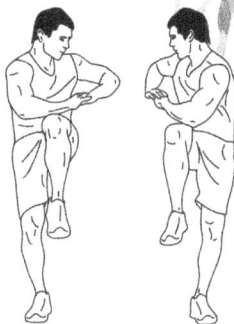

40 Split Lunges

Step into a lunge and go up, without moving off the spot, as illustrated. Repeat 40 times in total - 20 left side, 20 right side. Split into manageable sets.

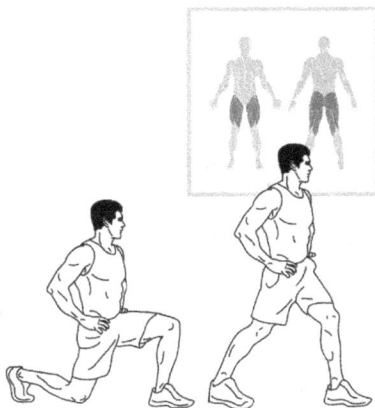

Extra Credit: 20/20 in one go

2 Minutes Wall-Sit

Set a timer and sit against the wall as illustrated. Hold it for 2 minutes in total. Split into manageable sets.

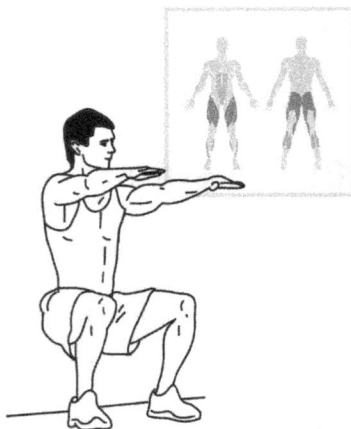

Extra Credit: in one go

187

2 Minutes Tree Pose

Hold the Tree Pose (as illustrated) for
60 seconds in one go, change sides
and hold it for another 60 seconds.

Extra Credit: in one go, keep balance

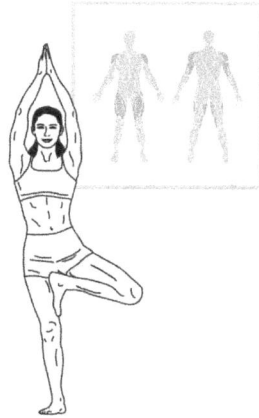

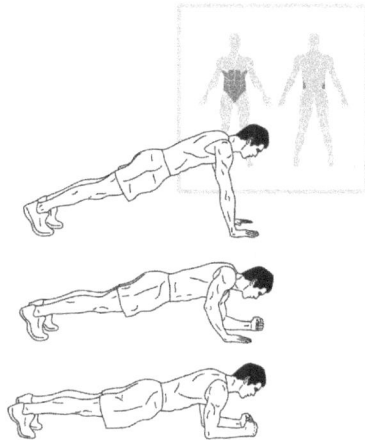

188

20 Up & Down Planks

Lower yourself from a plank into an
elbow plank - 20 times in total. All the
way down and all the way up is 1 rep.
Split into manageable sets.

Extra Credit: in one go,

keep the plank

189

15 Cross Tricep Extensions

Get into a plank position, hands crossed over each other. Lower yourself down until your elbows touch the floor = 15 times in total. Split into manageable sets.

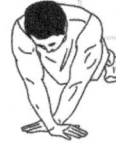

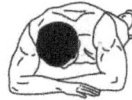

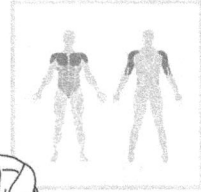

Extra Credit: in one go

190

60 Reverse Lunges

Step back into a lunge - 60 times in total. Split into manageable sets.

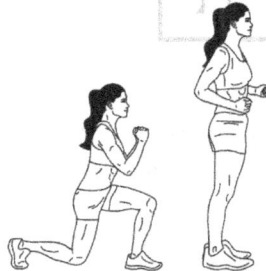

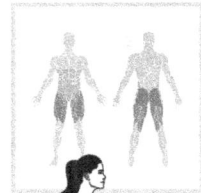

Extra Credit: in one go

40 Circle Crunches

Do crunches in a circular motion
as illustrated - 40 times in total, 20
crunches clockwise, 20 crunches
countercloclwise. Split into manageable sets.

Extra Credit: in one go

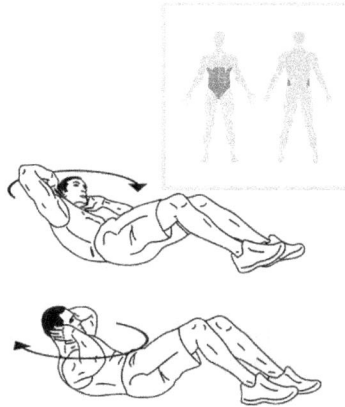

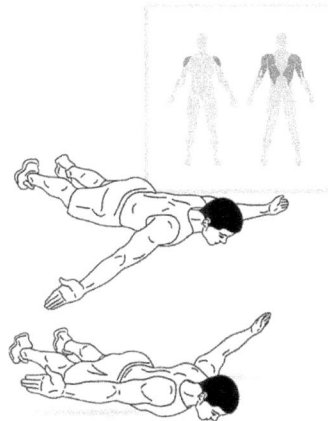

40 Prone Reverse Fly

Lie on the floor face down, arms
extended to your sides, thumbs
pointed upwards. Raise your arms
off the floor 40 times in total. Split
into manageable sets.

Extra Credit: in one go

193

200 Squat Hold Punches

Lower yourself into a squat, hold it and throw punches until you hit 200 punches in total.
Split into manageable sets.

Extra Credit: in one go

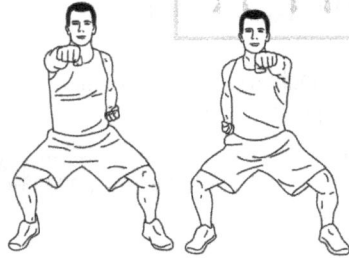

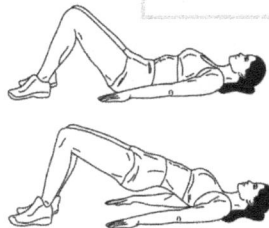

194

40 Bridges

Lie down, knees bent as illustrated and raise your hips off the floor = 40 times in total. Split into manageable sets.

Extra Credit: in one go

195

60 Seconds Plank Leg Raises

Set a timer and do plank leg raises
for 60 seconds in total;
Split into manageable sets. Change
legs halfway through.

Extra Credit: in one go

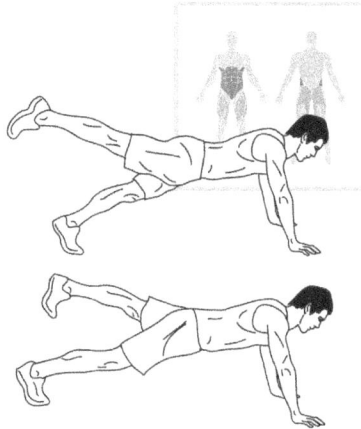

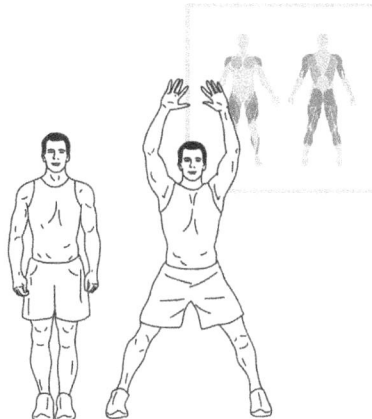

196

70 Jumping Jacks

Do jumping jacks until you hit 70
in total. Split into manageable sets.

Extra Credit: in one go

197

15 Sky Diver Push-Ups

Get into a plank position and drop
down so your chest rests on the
floor, raise your arms up as illustrated. Push back up. repeat 15 times in
total.

Extra Credit: in one go

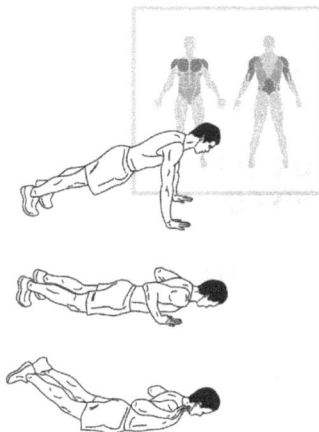

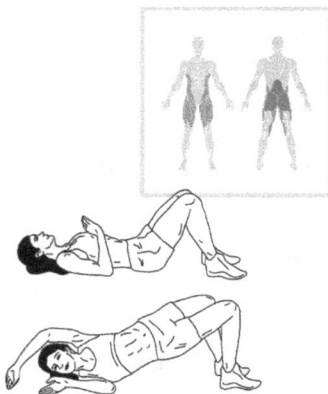

198

40 Bridge Taps

Lie down, raise your hips up and tap
the floor over your head. Repeat 40
times in total. Split into manageable
sets.

Extra Credit: in one go

199

15 Jump Knee Tucks

Jump up bringing your knees to your chest - 15 times in total.
Split into manageable sets.

Extra Credit: in one go

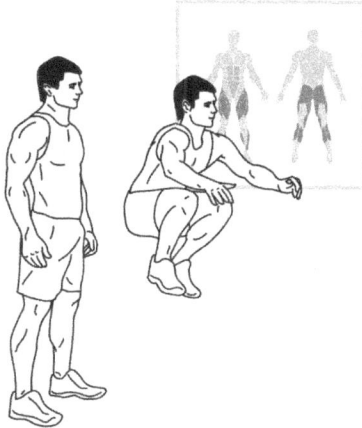

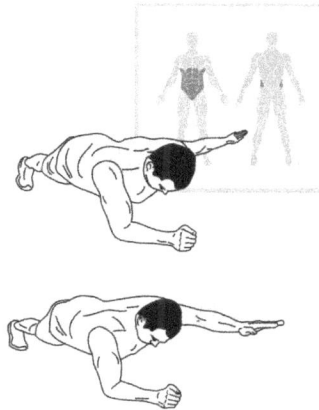

200

40 Seagulls

Get into an elbow plank, stretch your hand in front of you and move it to the side. Repeat until you hit 40 reps in total. Split into manageable sets.

Extra Credit: in one go

30 Raised Leg Circles

Get down on the floor and raise your legs at roughly 45 degrees. "Draw" circles in the air - 30 in total. Split into manageable sets.

Extra Credit: in one go

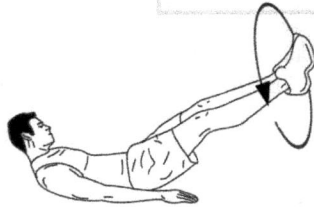

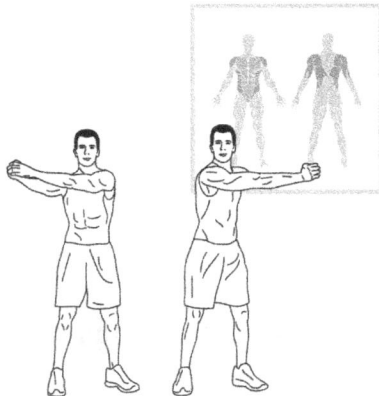

80 Side-to-Side Chops

"Chop" side to side, as illustrated, until you hit 80 chops in total. Split into manageable sets.

Extra Credit: in one go

203

100 W-Arm Extensions

Raise your arms up and then lower them down until your elbows are at shoulder level - as illustrated. Repeat 100 times in total. Split into manageable sets.

Extra Credit: in one go

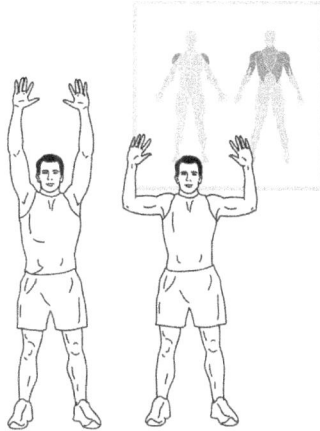

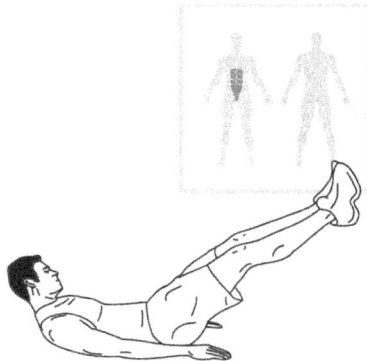

204

2 Minutes Raised Leg Hold

Set a timer, lie down and raise your legs at 45 degrees. Hold them up for 2 minutes in total.

Extra Credit: in one go

80 Seal Jacks

Start with your arms raised to
your sides, legs wide then jump in,
bringing your hands together.
Repeat 80 times in total.

Extra Credit: in one go

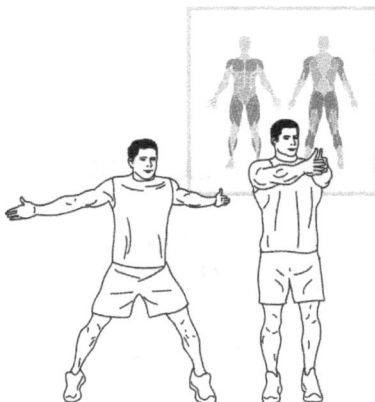

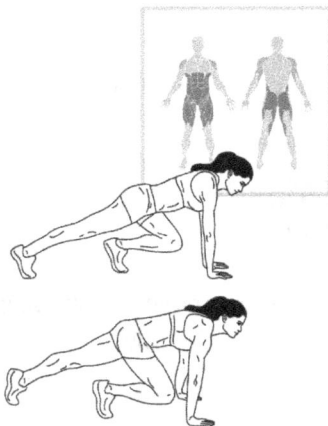

100 Climbers

Get down into a plank. Begin to climb
on the spot, as fast as you can, until
you hit 100 reps in total (50 per leg).
Split into manageable sets.

Extra Credit: in one go

207

40 Plank Rotations

Get into a plank and do rotations as illustrated until you hit 40 in total. Split into manageable sets.

Extra Credit: in one go

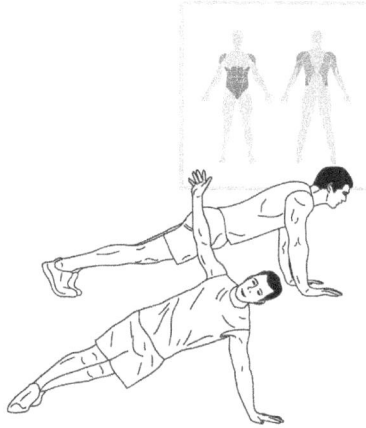

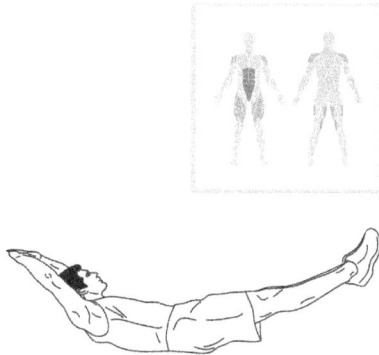

208

60 Seconds Hollow Hold

Stretch out, raise your arms and legs off the floor as illustrated. Hold it for 60 seconds in total. Split into manageable sets.

Extra Credit: in one go

209

2 Minutes O-Pose Hold

Set a timer, sit down on the floor, lift your feet and arms up as illustrated and hold the pose for 2 minutes in total. Split into manageable sets.

Extra Credit: in one go

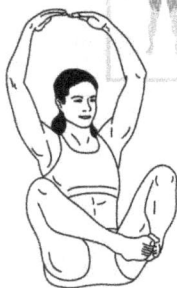

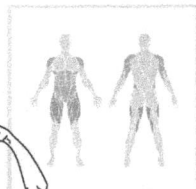

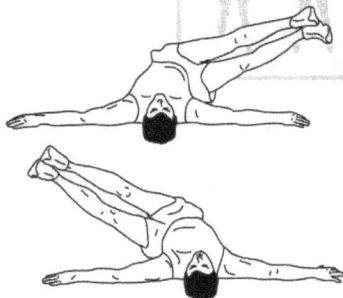

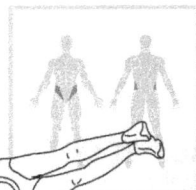

210

30 Windshield Wipers

Lie down on the floor or a bed, raise your legs up at 90 degrees. Tilt them to the left and then tilt them to the right (= 2 reps) 30 times in total.

Extra Credit: in one go

40 Reverse Plank Kicks

Get into a reverse plank, bring your
knee in and push your foot away
40 times in total; 20 on the left leg,
20 on the right leg.

Extra Credit: 20 / 20 in one go

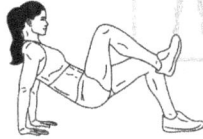

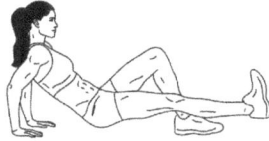

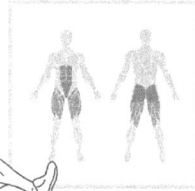

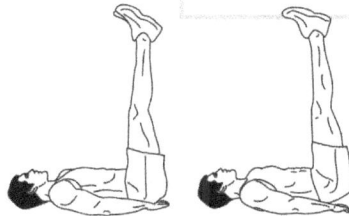

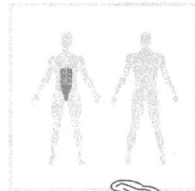

40 Pulse Ups

Lie down, raise your legs up at a 90
degrees angle and lift your hips off
the floor slightly. Pulse up and down
as illustrated 40 times in total.

Extra Credit: in one go

20 Push-Up + Jab + Cross

Drop into a push-up then jump up and throw a jab followed up by a cross. Repeat until you hit 20 in total. Split into manageable sets.

Extra Credit: in one go

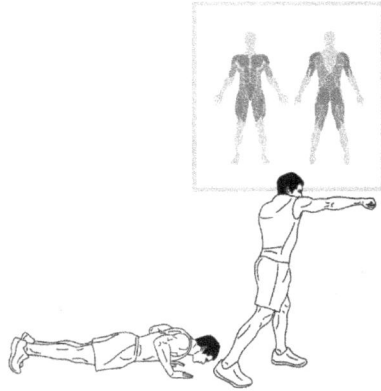

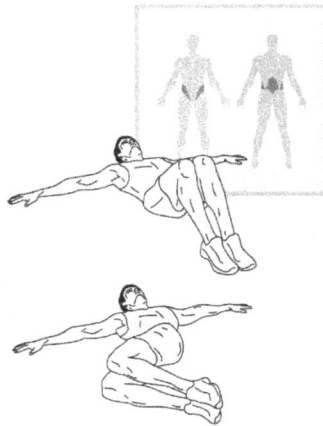

50 Knee Rolls

Lie down, knees bent as illustrated. Roll them from side to side, until they touch the floor - 50 times in total. Split into manageable sets.

Extra Credit: in one go

80 Shoulder Taps

Get into a plank position and tap your
left shoulder - 40 times, then tap
your right houlder 40 times;
80 times in total.

Extra Credit: in one go, keep the
plank

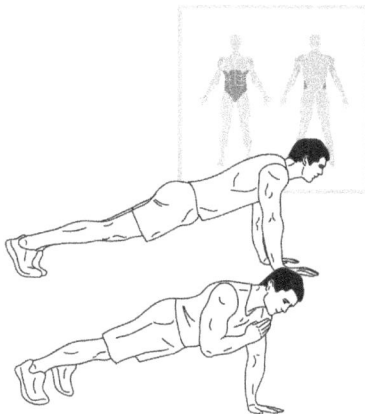

2 Minutes Calf Raise Hold

Set a timer and stand on tip toe for
2 minutes in total.
Split into manageable sets.

Extra Credit: in one go, heels not
touching the floor

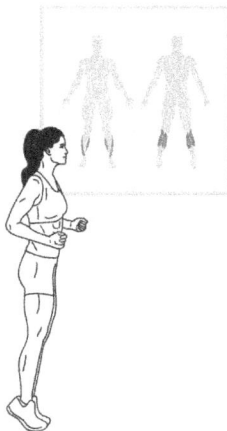

217

2 Minutes Skiers

Set a timer and do skiers, as illustrated for 2 minutes in total. Split into manageable sets.

Extra Credit: in one go

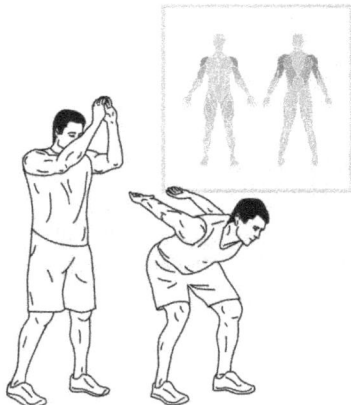

218

2 Minutes Chest Squeeze

Stand upright with both arms out in front of you, bent at a 90 degree angle. Lock your hands together and squeeze as hard as you can. Hold the contraction for 2 minutes in total.

Extra Credit: non-stop

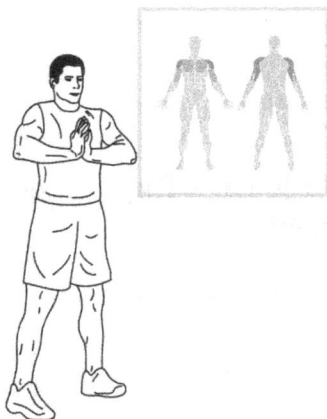

40 Sit-Ups

Lie down on the floor and do sit-ups until you hit 40 in total. Split into manageable sets.

Extra Credit: in one go

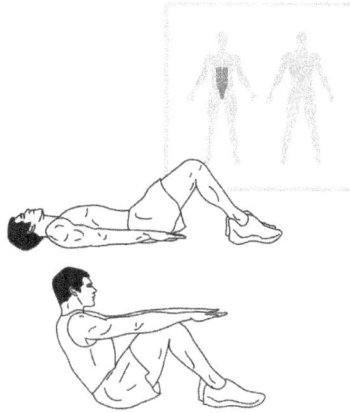

30 Single Leg Deadlifts

Start standing on left leg with right leg lifted and bent at a 90-degree angle in front of body. Bend forward, hands reaching toward the floor as right leg extends directly behind the body. Repeat 30 times in total, 15 per side.

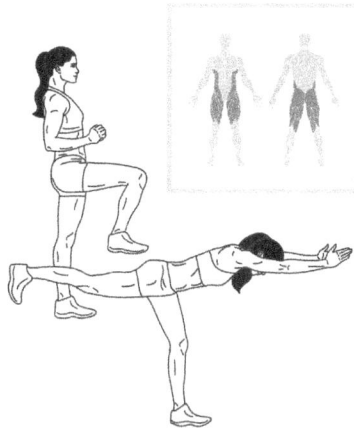

Extra Credit: 15/15, in one go

40 Infinity Circles

Raise your leg to the side, waist
height and draw infinity symbol in
the air - 40 in total, 20 each leg. Split
into manageable sets.

Extra Credit: in one go

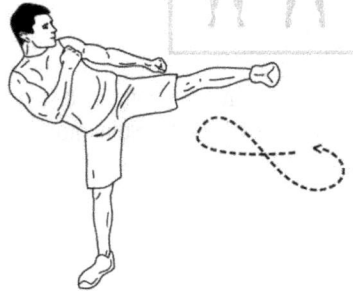

3 Minutes Hops on the Spot

Set a timer and bounce on the spot
(two feet) for 3 minutes in total. Try
to keep pauses to a minimum.

Extra Credit: non-stop

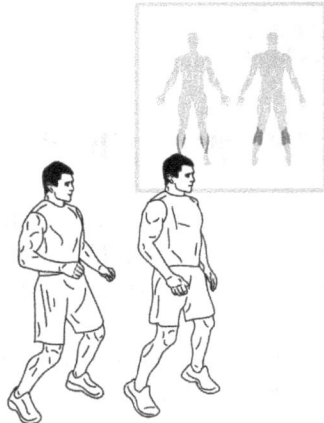

223

30 Glute Flex

Lie down on your stomach, legs bent at 90 degrees, heels together. Raise your buttocks off the flor as high as you can - 30 times in total.

Extra Credit: in one go

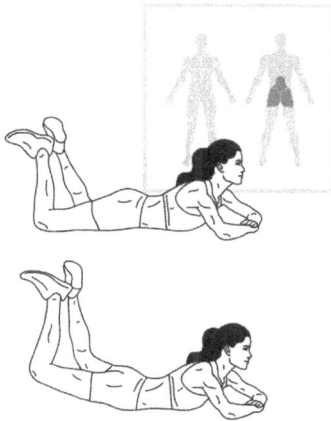

224

80 Leg Extensions

Get on your hands and knees and raise your left leg up bent at 90 degrees - continue until you hit 40 repetitions in total; switch legs halfway and do another 40. Split into manageable sets.

Extra Credit: 40/40, in one go

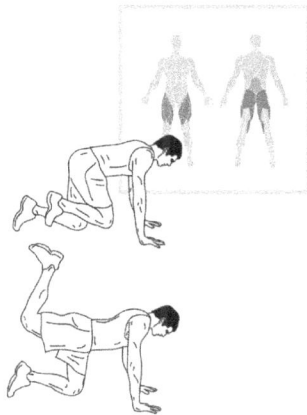

16 Archer Push-Ups

Get into a plank, one arm extended
away from you and do 16 push-ups
in total. Split into manageable sets.
Switch sides with every rep.

Extra Credit: in one go

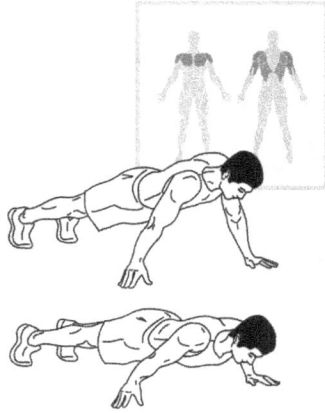

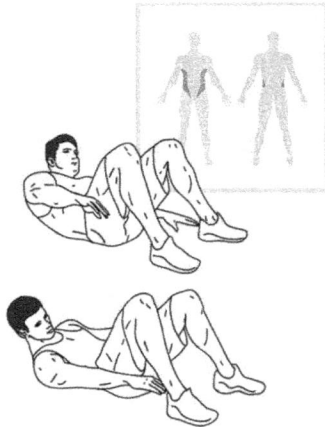

60 Heel Taps

Lie down on the floor as illustrated,
reach for, and then tap your heels
- 60 times in total. Split into
manageable sets.

Extra Credit: in one go

227

3 Minutes Leg Raise Hold

Lie down on the floor on your side and raise your leg at about 30 degrees - as illustrated. Hold it up for 3 minutes in total, 90 seconds per side. Split into manageable sets.

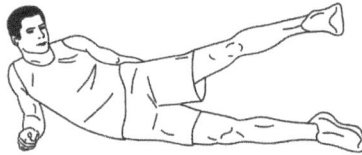

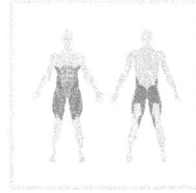

Extra Credit: in one go

228

60 Squat + Step Back

Lower yourself into a deep squat and place your hands on your knees so your elbows point to your sides as illustrated, then step back - 60 times in total. Split into manageable sets.

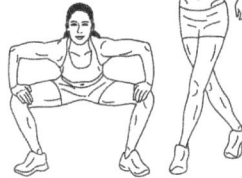

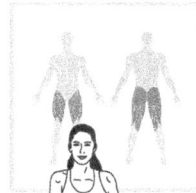

Extra Credit: in one go

229

40 Side Plank Rotations

Get into a side elbow plank, slide your hand under your torso and bring it up towards the ceiling as illustrated. 20 left side, 20 right side = 40 times in total. Split into manageable sets.

Extra Credit: in one go

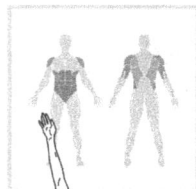

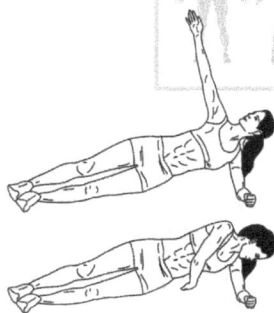

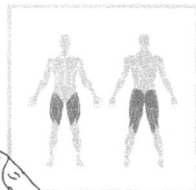

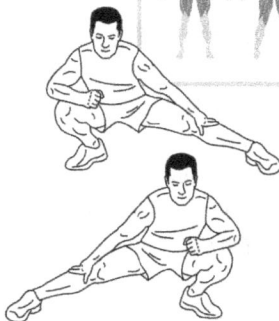

230

60 Side-To-Side Lunges

Get into a deep side lunge position and shift your body to the other side without standing up, 60 times in total. Split into manageable sets.

Extra Credit: in one go

231

30 Side V-Ups

Lie down on your side, legs extended straight, one arm behind your head. Fold your body up (into a V) so your elbow touches your knee - 30 times in total. Split into manageable sets.

Extra Credit: 15/15, in one go

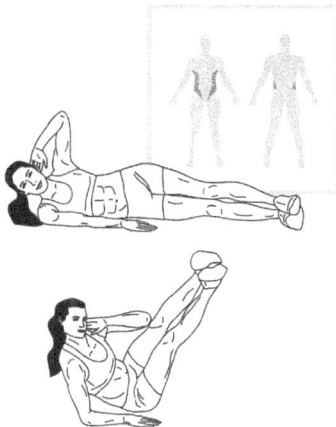

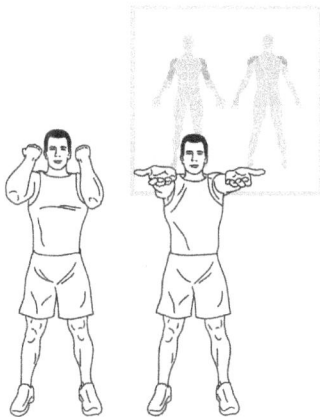

232

100 Bicep Extensions

Bring your arms to your ears and unroll them out palm outwards, as illustrated, 100 times in total. Split into manageable sets.

Extra Credit: in one go

233

100 Side Leg Raises

Raise your right leg to your side at 90 degrees until you hit 50 reps; change legs and do another 50, 100 in total. You can hold on to something.

Extra Credit: 50/50 in one go

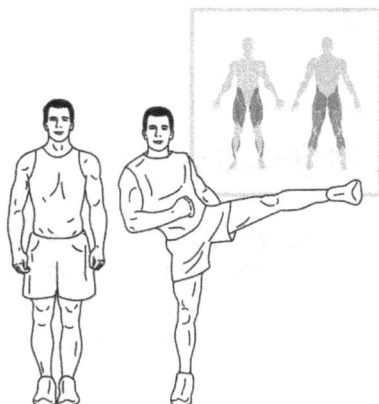

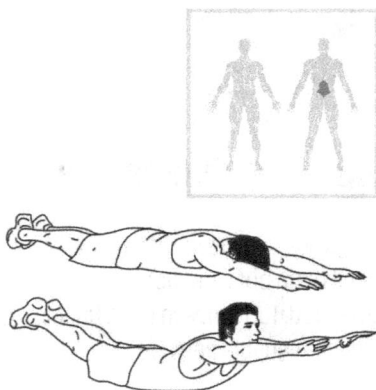

234

30 Superman Extensions

Lie down on the floor, stretch your arms in front of you and do superman extensions as illustrated. Split into manageable sets.

Extra Credit: in one go

40 Crunch Kicks

Sit down on the floor as illustrated, raise your legs up at roughly 45 degrees and do crunch kicks - 40 in total. Split into manageable sets.

Extra Credit: in one go, don't lower your legs down

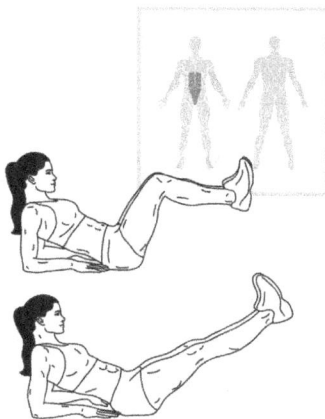

2 Minutes Raised Arm Circles

Set a timer, raise your arms up shoulder height and rotate them for 2 minutes in total. Split into manageable sets.

Extra Credit: non-stop

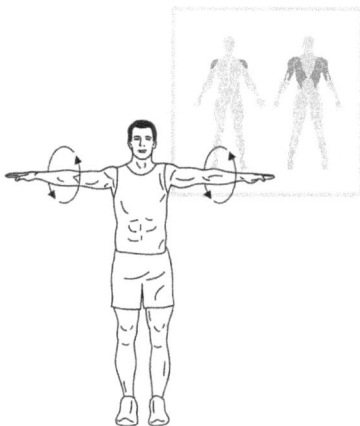

237

30 Plank Jacks

Do squats until you hit 30 in total.
Split into manageabe sets - as fewer
as possible.

Extra Credit: in one go

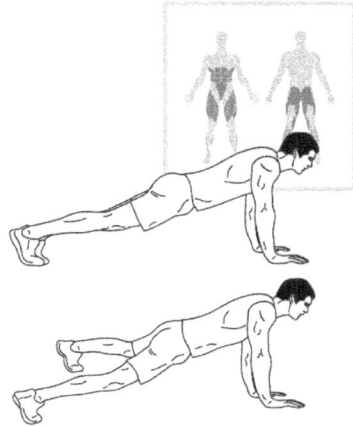

238

3 Minutes March Steps

Set a timer and do march steps
(march on the spot) for 3 minutes in
total. Split into manageable sets.

Extra Credit: non-stop

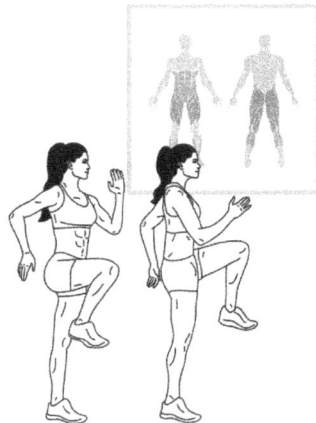

20 Basic Burpees With a Jump

Do basic burpees with a jump (no push-up) as fast as you can until you hit 20 in total. Split into manageable sets.

Extra Credit: in one go

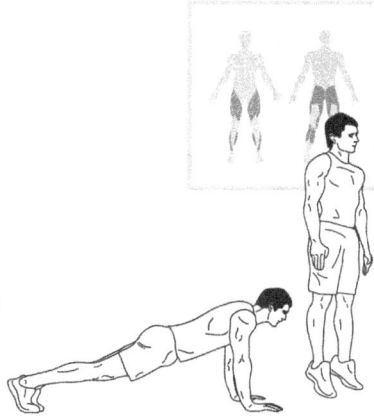

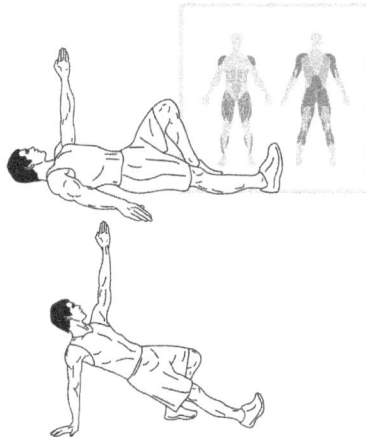

50 Get-Ups

Sit down on the floor, lean on one arm and hold the other extended above your shoulder. Liift yourself up as illustrated - 50 times in total. Split into manageable sets.

Extra Credit: in one go

50 Knee-to-Elbow Crunches

Get on the floor, place your hands behind your head and bring the opposite knee to opposite elbow 50 times in total.

Extra Credit: in one go

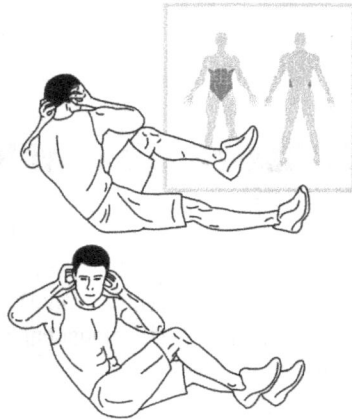

300 Overhead Punches

Do overhead punches, 150 with the right arm, 150 with the left arm, 300 times in total. Complete one side first before starting on the other. Split into manageable sets.

Extra Credit: 150/150, in one go

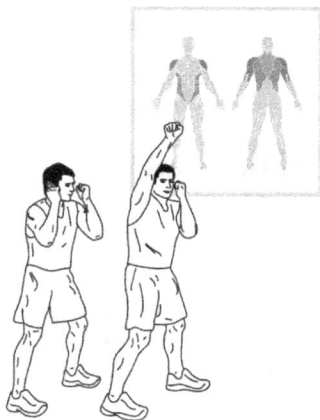

60 Front Kicks

Do front kicks until you hit 60 in total.
Split into manageable sets.

Extra Credit: 30/30, in one go
Extra Extra Credit: foot not touching
the floor

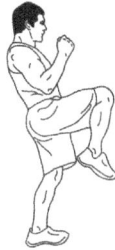

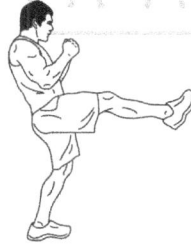

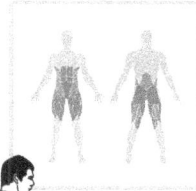

3 Minutes Meditation

Set a timer and meditate for 3
minutes in total. Relax. Keep cool.
Breathe.

Extra Credit: in one go

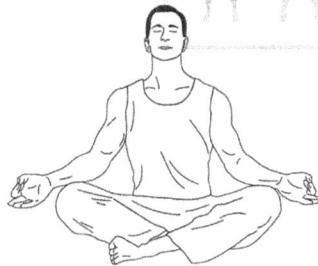

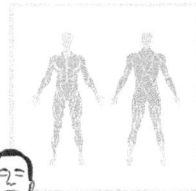

60 Lunge Step-Ups

Start from a lunge and step up 60
times in total, 30 times per side
(complete one side first, then the
other). Split into manageable sets.

Extra Credit: in one go

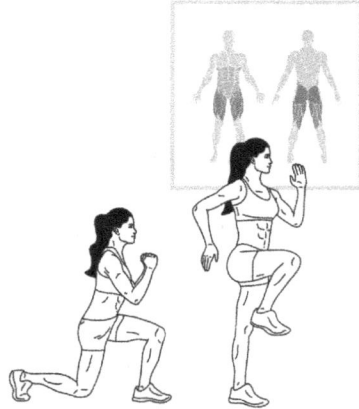

60 Seconds Flutter Kicks

Set a timer and do flutter kicks as
fast as you can for 60 seconds in
total. Split into manageable sets.

Extra Credit: non-stop

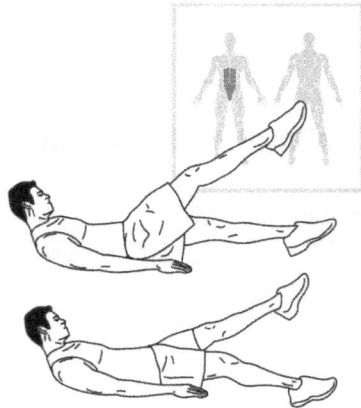

247

10 Pop-Ups

Kneel on the floor, sitting back on heels. Raise arms overhead, then throw arms back behind body before driving them forward and explosively popping up off knees to land on feet. Perform a tuck jump - 10 times in total.

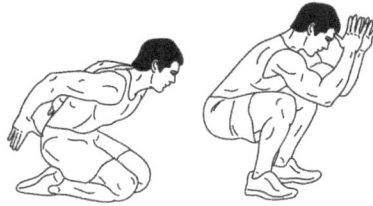

Extra Credit: in one go

248

40 Sitting Twists

Sit down on the floor or a sofa and do sitting twists, as illustrated - 40 in total. Split into manageable sets.

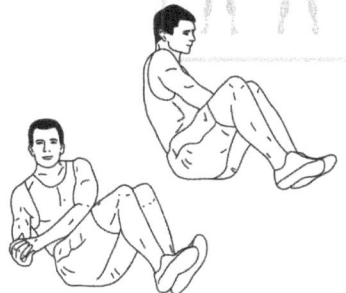

Extra Credit: in one go

249

20 Plank Walk-Outs

Walk out into a plank, as illustrated, until you hit 20 in total. Split into manageable sets.

Extra Credit: in one go

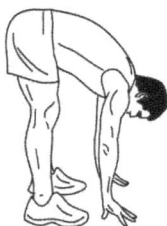

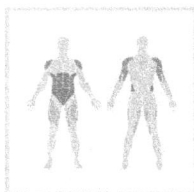

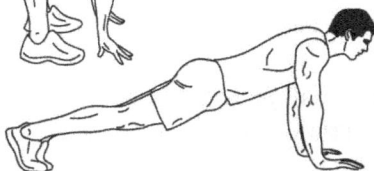

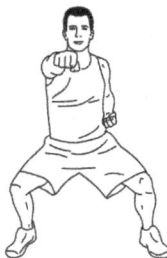

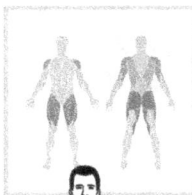

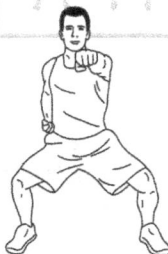

250

200 Squat Hold Punches

Lower yourself into a squat, hold it and throw punches until you hit 200 punches in total.
Split into manageable sets.

Extra Credit: in one go

251

30 Swipers

Get on the floor into a relaxed
table position and do swipers,
as illustrated, 30 times in total.
Split into manageable sets.

Extra Credit: in one go

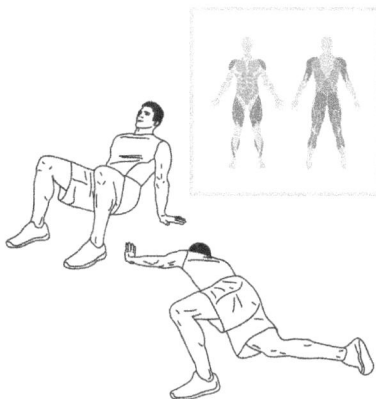

252

50 Split Lunges

Step into a lunge and go up, without
moving off the spot, as illustrated.
Repeat 40 times in total- 25 left side,
25 right side. Split into manageable
sets.

Extra Credit: 25/25 in one go

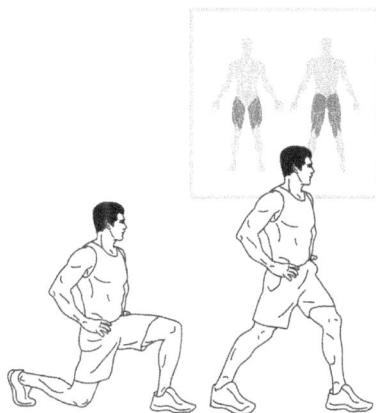

40 Butterfly Dips

Sit down on the floor and lean back, heels together. Lift yourself up bringing your knees together. Repeat 40 times in total. Split into manageable sets.

Extra Credit: in one go

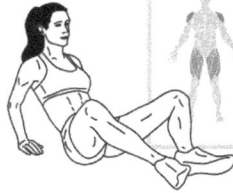

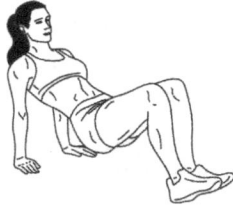

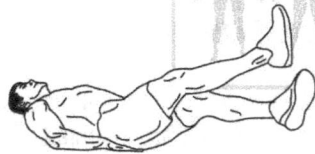

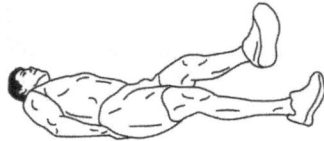

50 Scissors

Lie down, raise your legs at roughly 30 degrees off the floor and do scissors in the air until you hit 50 reps, cross over & under = 2 reps.

Extra Credit: in one go

40 Lunges With Twist

Raise your arms in front of you and step forward into a lunge, twisting your body to the side. Repeat 40 times in total. Split into manageable sets.

Extra Credit: 20/20, in one go

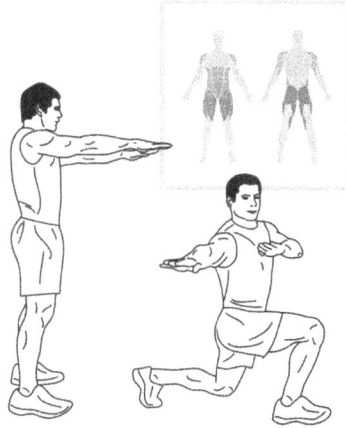

50 Balance Back Kicks

Balance on one leg and kick back with the other as illustrated - 50 times in total; 25 per leg.

Extra Credit: 25/25, in one go

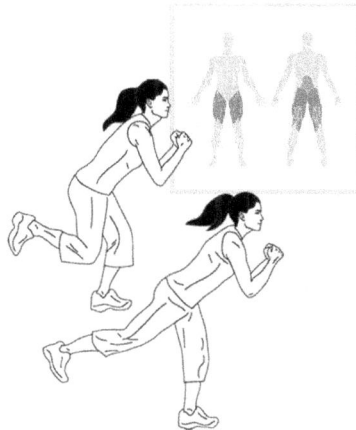

257

30 Seconds Push-Up Plank Hold

Get into a plank and lower yourself down into a push-up - hold it for 30 seconds in total.

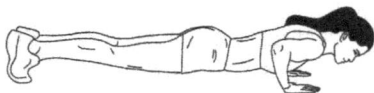

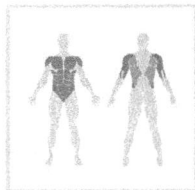

Extra Credit: in one go

258

50 Squat Hops on the Spot

Place your hands behind your head and lower yourself into a deep squat. Hop on the spot, without getting up, 50 times in total. Split into manageable sets.

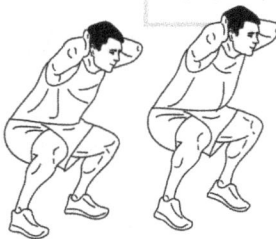

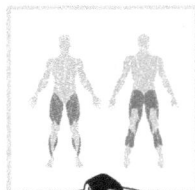

Extra Credit: in one go

259

20 Sky Diver Push-Ups

Get into a plank position and drop down so your chest rests on the floor, raise your arms up as illustrated. Push back up. repeat 20 times in total.

Extra Credit: in one go

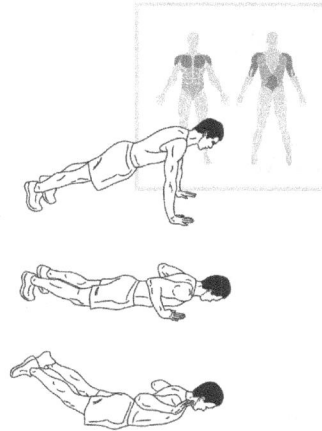

260

40 Single Leg Deadlifts

Start standing on left leg with right leg lifted and bent at a 90-degree angle in front of body. Bend forward, hands reaching toward the floor as right leg extends directly behind the body. Repeat 40 times in total, 20 per side.

Extra Credit: 15/15, in one go

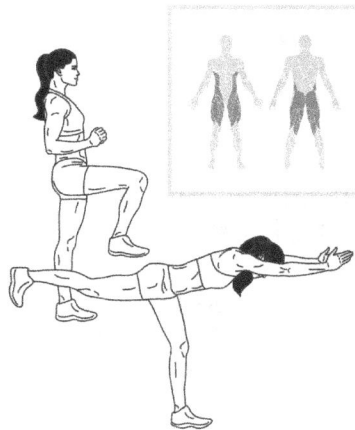

120 Climbers

Get down into a plank. Begin to climb on the spot, as fast as you can, until you hit 120 reps in total (60 per leg). Split into manageable sets.

Extra Credit: in one go

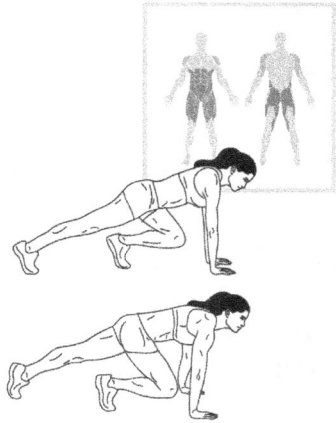

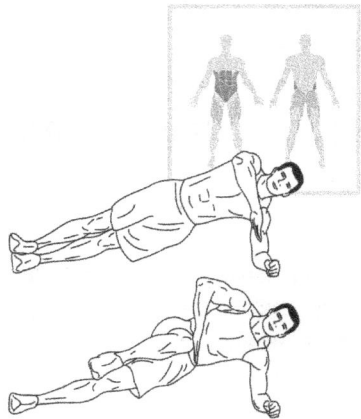

40 Side Plank Knee Taps

Get into a side plank and tap your knee 20 times. Change sides and do another 20 taps, 40 taps in total. Split into manageable sets.

Extra Credit: in one go

2 Minutes Tricep Dip Hold

Lower yourself into a tricep dip and hold it for 2 minutes in total. Split into manageable sets.

Extra Credit: in one go

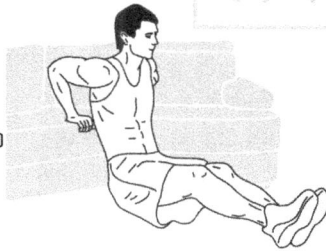

3 Minutes Butt Kicks

Set a timer and do butt kicks for 3 minutes in total. Split into manageable sets.

Extra Credit: non-stop

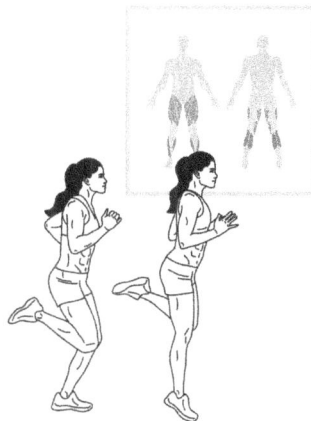

30 Reverse Crunches

Lie down on the floor, legs bent
at roughly 90 degrees. Roll your
lower body up towards your chest
as illustrated - 30 times in total. Split
into manageable sets.

Extra Credit: in one go

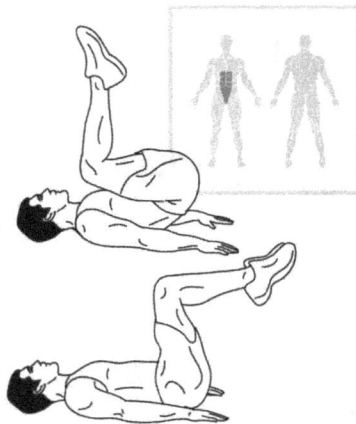

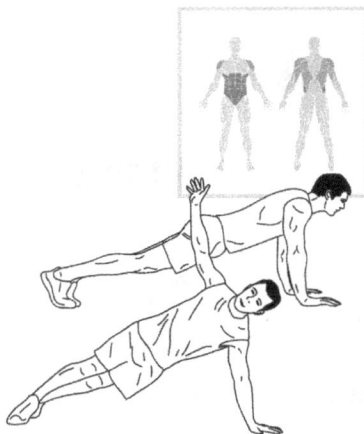

50 Plank Rotations

Get into a plank and do rotations as
illustrated until you hit 50 in total.
Split into manageable sets.

Extra Credit: in one go

30 Hop Heel Clicks

Hop up and click your heels - 30 times in total. Split into manageable sets.

Extra Credit: in one go

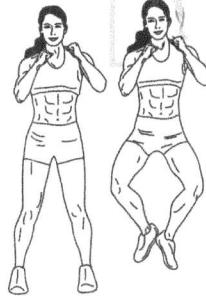

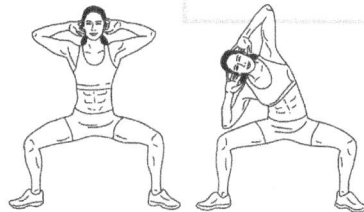

50 Squat Hold Side Bends

Lower yourself into a squat and place your arms behind your head, as illustrated. Bend to the side and reach with your elbow to your knee - 50 times in total. Split into manageable sets.

Extra Credit: in one go

15 Diamond Push-Ups

Get into a plank position, bring your
hands together forming a "diamond"
and do push-ups - 15 in total. Split
into manageable sets.

Extra Credit: in one go

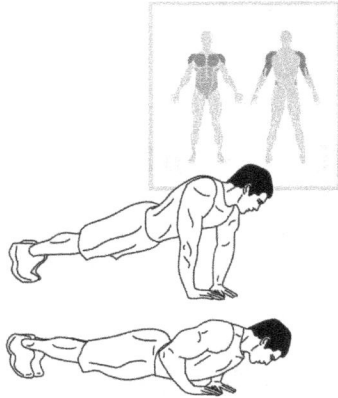

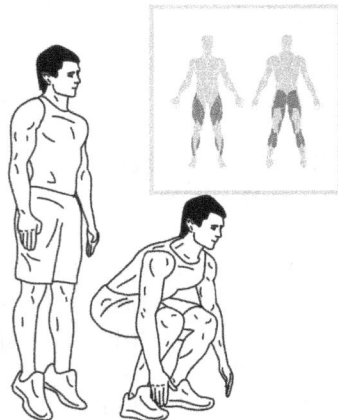

20 Jump Squats

Do jump squats until you hit 20 in
total. Split into manageable sets.

Extra Credit: in one go

2 Minutes Clench / Unclench

Set a timer then clench and unclench your hands as fast as you can for 2 minutes in total. Split into manageable sets.

Extra Credit: non-stop

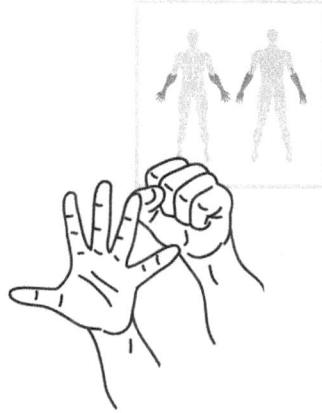

80 March Twists

March on the spot while twisting so your opposite elbow touches your opposite knee, as illustrated - 80 times in total.

Extra Credit: in one go

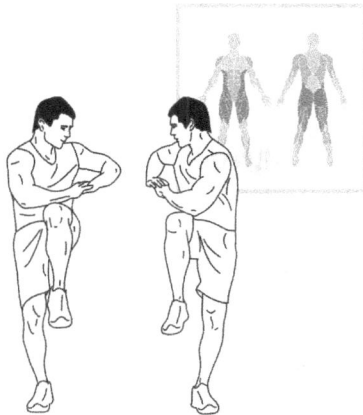

273

40 Forward Lunges

Step into a forward lunge 40 times in total. Split into manageable sets.

Extra Credit: in one go

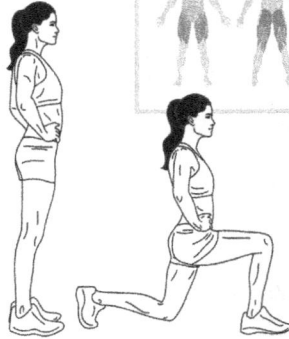

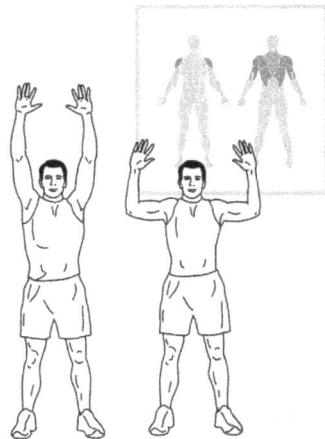

274

120 W-Arm Extensions

Raise your arms up and then lower them down until your elbows are at shoulder level - as illustrated. Repeat 120 times in total. Split into manageable sets.

Extra Credit: in one go

275

2 Minutes Toe Tap Hops

Set a timer, hop up and tap your opposite toe with the opposite hand, as fast as you can, for 2 minutes in total. Split into manageable sets.

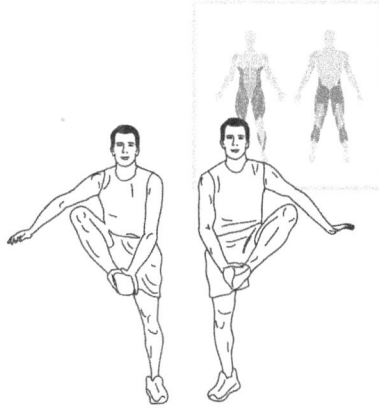

Extra Credit: in one go

276

40 Infinity Circles

Lie down and raise your legs at 90 degrees as illustrated. "Draw" an infinity symbol in the air with your feet - 40 times in total. Split into manageable sets.

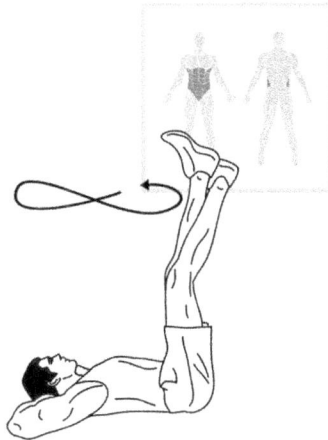

Extra Credit: in one go

277

50 Plank
Knee-to-Elbows

Bring opposite knee to opposite
elbow while in a knee-plank -
50 times in total, 25 times per side.
Complete one side first, then the
other. Split into manageable sets.

Extra Credit: in one go

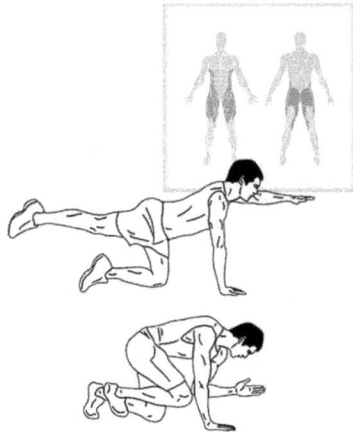

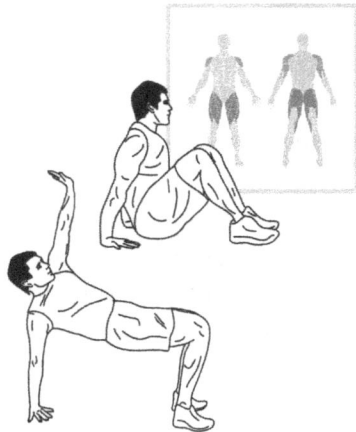

278

40 Full Bridge Reach

Get into a full bridge position, as
illustrated, reach towards the ceiling
with your left hand and then with
your right hand - 40 times in total.
Split into manageable sets.

Extra Credit: in one go

20 Raised Leg Push-Ups

Get into a plank position and raise your left leg, lower yourself down and then push yourself up - 20 times in total. Switch legs every time Split into manageable sets.

Extra Credit: in one go

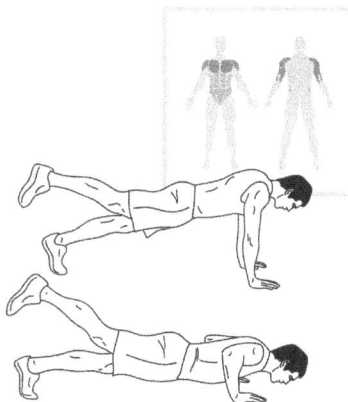

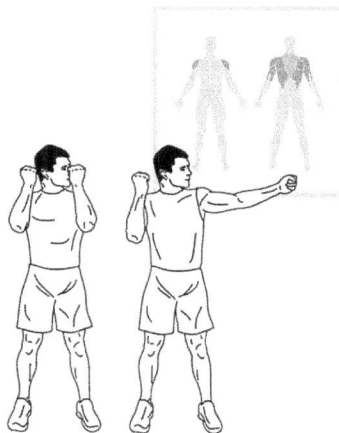

200 Backfists

Throw backfists to the right until you hit 100, change sides and throw backfists to the left - another 100; 200 times in total. Split into manageable sets.

Extra Credit: in one go

40 High Crunches

Lie down on the floor, stretch your arms above you towards the ceiling and do crunches as illustrated - 40 in total. Split into manageable sets.

Extra Credit: in one go

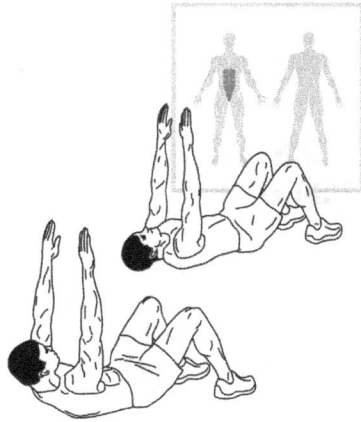

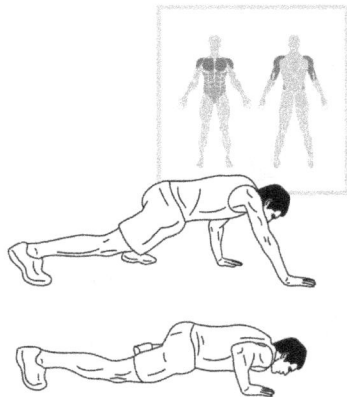

20 Dragon Push-Ups

Get into a plank, step in as illustrated and do a push-up, 20 in total. Split into manageable sets. Change legs each time.

Extra Credit: in one go

283

60 Seconds Pacer Steps

Set a timer and lower yourself into a squat. Pace on the spot while in a squat position as fast as you can - 60 seconds in total.

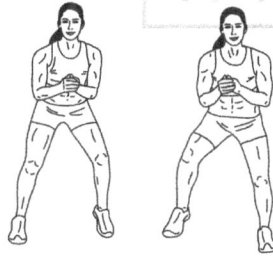

Extra Credit: in one go

284

50 Dead Bugs

Lay down on the floor with your hands extended above you toward the ceiling. Bend your knees in 90 degree angle. Slowly lower the opposite arm and the opposite leg down to the floor simultaneously. Repeat 50 times in total.

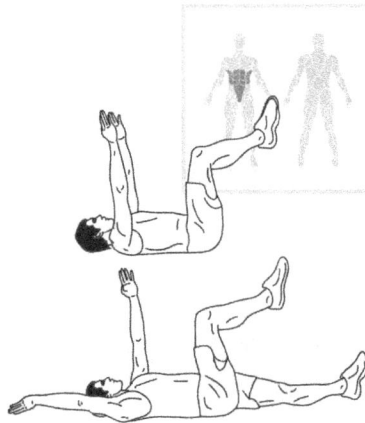

Extra Credit: in one go

285

100 Side-to-Side Chops

"Chop" side to side, as illustrated, until you hit 100 chops in total. Split into manageable sets.

Extra Credit: in one go

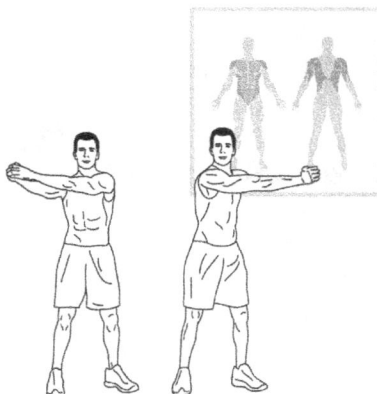

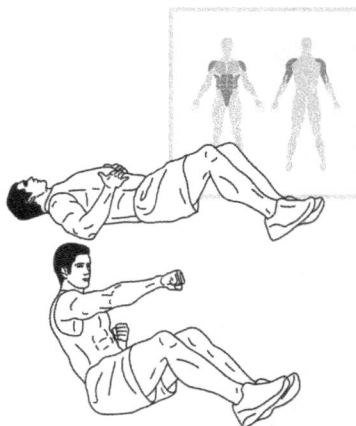

286

40 Sit-Up Punches

Sit up and throw a jab and a cross (2 punches). Repeat until you hit 40 sit-up punches in total. Split into manageable sets.

Extra Credit: in one go

287

2 Minutes Knee Strikes

Set a timer and do knee strikes for 2 minutes in total. Split into manageable sets.

Extra Credit: non-stop

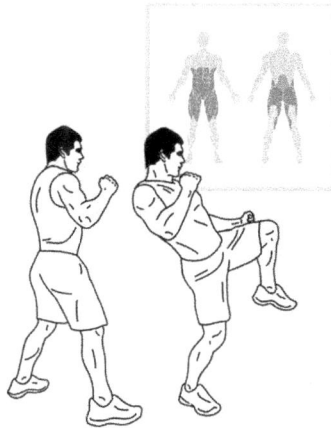

288

20 L-Sit Ups

Lie down on the floor, arms raised overhead. Sit up while keeping your arms still over your head, as illustrated. Split into manageable sets.

Extra Credit: in one go

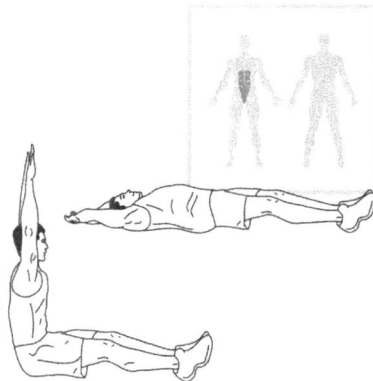

60 Seconds Back Arch Balance Hold

Get on the floor and grab your opposite ankle with the opposite hand as illustrated. Hold the pose for 30 seconds per side, 60 Seconds in total. Split into manageable sets.

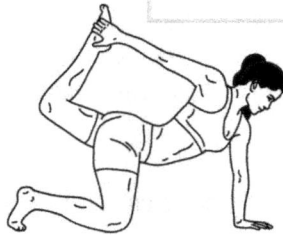

Extra Credit: in one go

10 Circle Push-Ups

Start in a plank position, tilt your body to the left in a half circle motion and do lower yourself into a push-up. Tilt your body to the right as you come up. Repeat 10 times in total. Split into manageable sets.

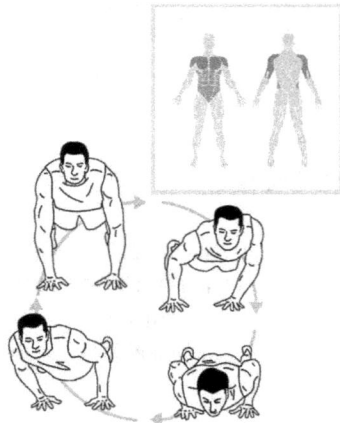

Extra Credit: in one go

291

20 Pop-Up Tripods

Balance on your hands as you pop your lower body up, straighten your legs and pop up. Land with your feet spread wide. Then jump back into a crouch. Repeat 20 times in total; split into manageable sets.

Extra Credit: in one go

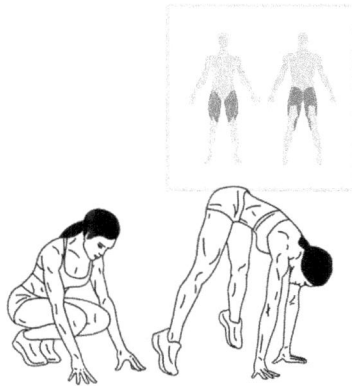

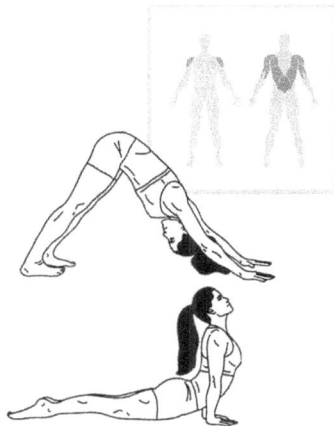

292

20 Downward Upward Dogs

Start from the downward dog position and slowly roll into an upward dog - 20 times in total. Split into manageable sets.

Extra Credit: in one go

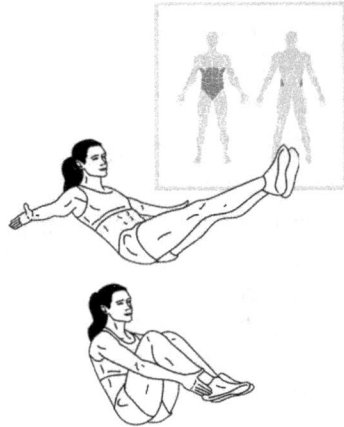

30 Boat Folds

Sit down on the floor, arms and legs lifted up as illustrated. Fold in and reach for your heels - 30 times in total. Split into manageable sets.

Extra Credit: in one go ,

keep your balance

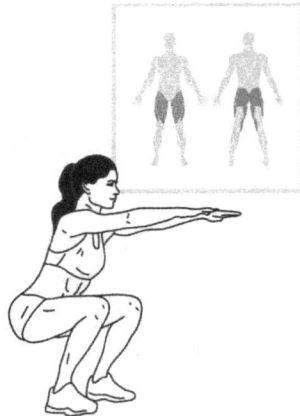

2 Minutes Squat Hold

Lower yourself into a squat (your glutes should be parallel to the floor) and hold it for 2 minutes in total. Split into manageable sets.

Extra Credit: in one go

295

50 Thigh Taps

Get into a plank position and tap your thighs - 50 times in total.
Split into manageable sets.

Extra Credit: in one go

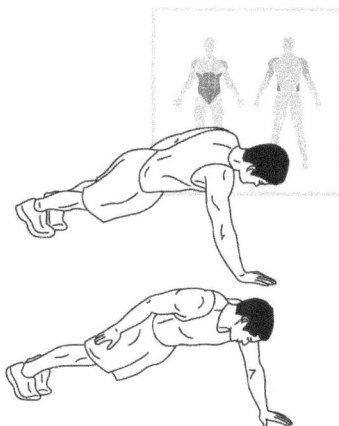

296

50 Single-Leg Bridges

Lie down on the floor, raise one leg up as illustrated. Lift your torso up - 50 times in total; 25 times per side. Split into manageable sets.

Extra Credit: 20 / 20, in one go

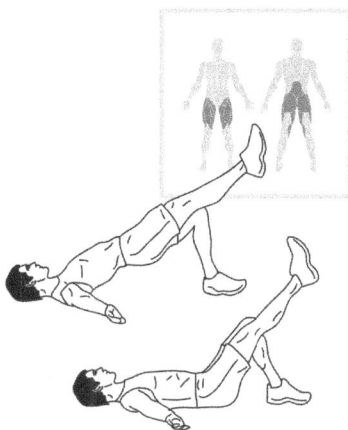

30 Forward Bends

Place your hands behind your head and bend forward. Repeat 30 times in total. Split into manageable sets.

Extra Credit: in one go

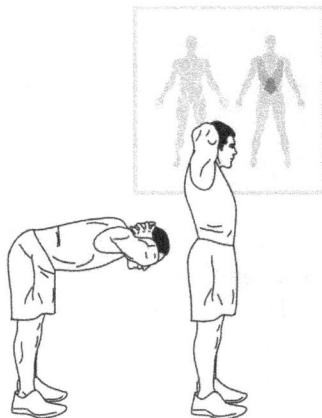

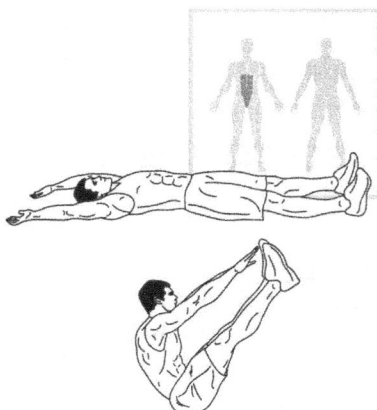

20 V-Ups

Lie down on the floor and fold into a V-Up, as illustrated, - 20 times in total. Split into manageable sets.

Extra Credit: in one go

299

50 Side Plank Rotations

Get into a side elbow plank, slide your hand under your torso and bring it up towards the ceiling as illustrated. 25 left side, 25 right side = 50 times in total. Split into manageable sets.

Extra Credit: in one go

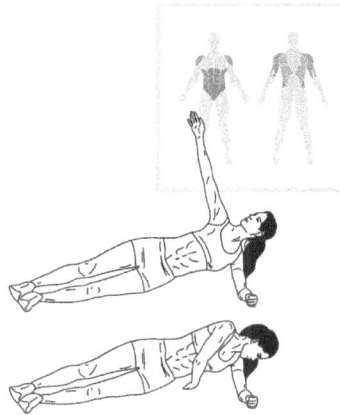

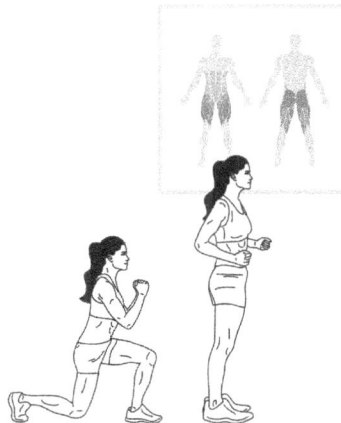

300

80 Reverse Lunges

Step back into a lunge - 80 times in total. Split into manageable sets.

Extra Credit: in one go

301

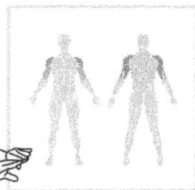

5 Minutes Raised Arms Hold

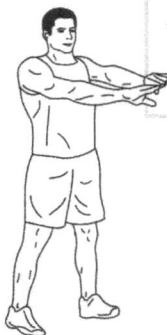

Set a timer and hold arms raised in front of you at shoulder height for 5 minutes in total. Split into manageable sets.

Extra Credit: in one go, keep arms up

302

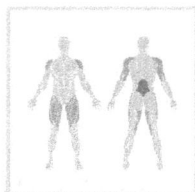

60 Seconds Swim

Lie down on your stomach and raise alternative arm and alternative leg off the floor as fast as you can. 60 seconds in total. Split into manageable sets.

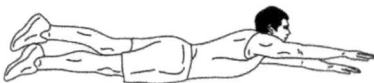

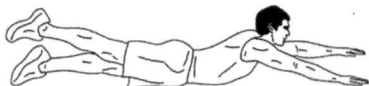

Extra Credit: in one go

2 minutes Elbow Plank Hold

Get on the floor and hold an elbow plank for 2 minutes in total. Split into manageable sets.

Extra Credit: in one go

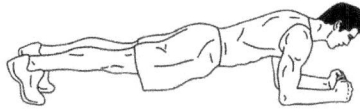

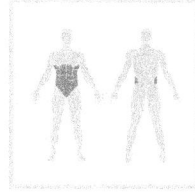

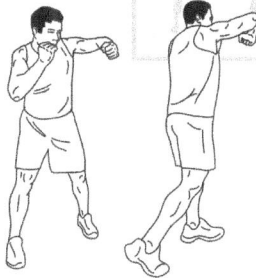

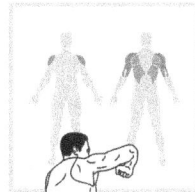

100 Hooks

Throw hooks until you hit 100 reps in total. Split into manageable sets.

Extra Credit: in one go

305

50 Prone Reverse Fly

Lie on the floor face down, arms
extended to your sides, thumbs
pointed upwards. Raise your arms
off the floor 50 times in total. Split
into manageable sets.

Extra Credit: in one go

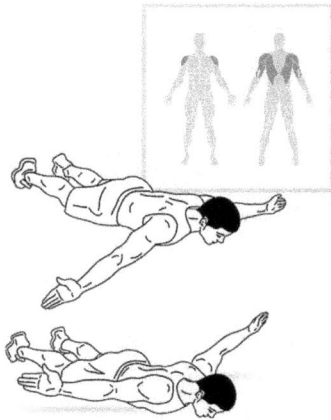

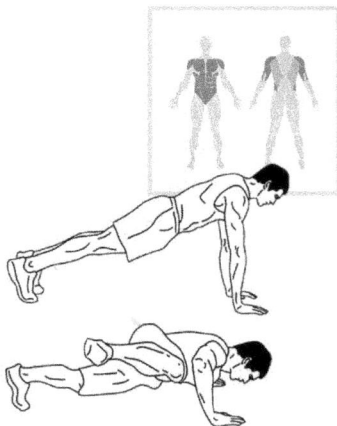

306

20 Push-Up Side Crunches

Get into a plank position and
lower yourself into a push-up while
bringing your knee to your elbow as
illustrated - 20 times in total.

Extra Credit: in one go

30 Roll-Ups

Sit down on the floor in a half sit-up, arms stretched out in front of you as illustrated. Roll up into a full sit-up - 30 times in total.

Extra Credit: in one go

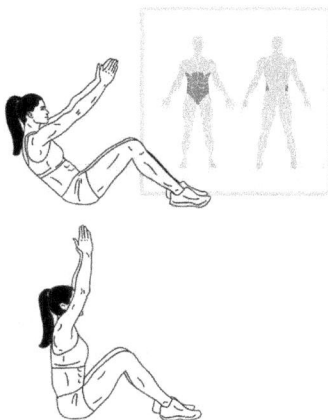

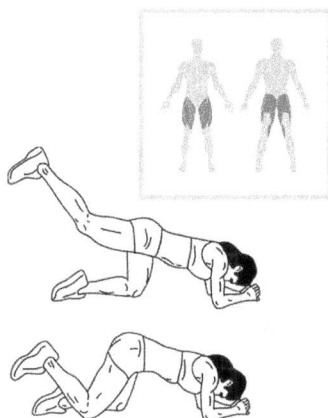

60 Back Kicks

Get on your elbows and knees and do back kicks, as illustrated. 30 times left leg, 30 times right leg - 60 times in total. Split into manageable sets.

Extra Credit: in one go

309

2 Minutes Sitting Down Leg Raises

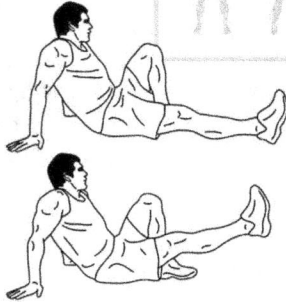

Set a timer and do sitting leg raises for 2 minutes in total. Change legs halfway through. Split into manageable sets.

Extra Credit: non-stop,

keep your leg up

310

60 Seconds Boat Pose Hold

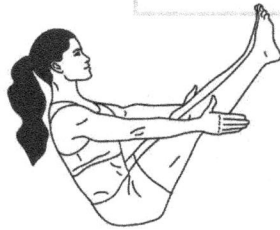

Hold a boat hold as illustrated for 60 seconds in total. Split into manageable sets.

Extra Credit: in one go

311

3 Minutes Wall-Sit

Set a timer and sit against the wall as illustrated. Hold it for 3 minutes in total. Split into manageable sets.

Extra Credit: in one go

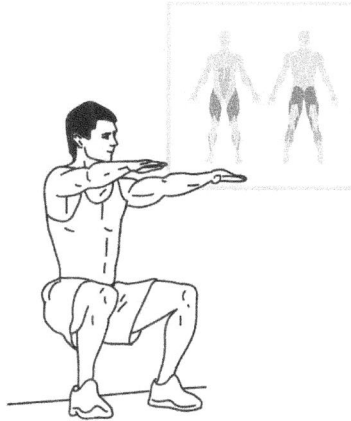

312

40 Scorpion Twists

Lie down on the floor, bend your right knee, and lift your right leg as high as you can then twist your hips and reach your right foot over to touch the ground on the outside of your left leg - 40 times in total; 20 times per side.

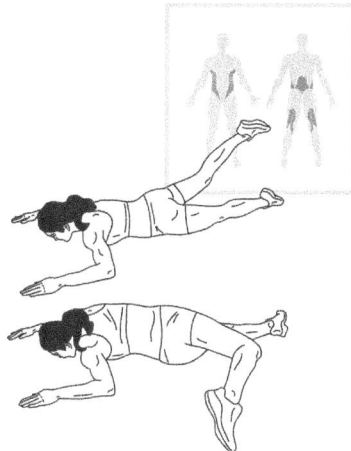

Extra Credit: in one go

313

4 Minutes Butt Kicks

Set a timer and do butt kicks for
4 minutes in total. Split into
manageable sets.

Extra Credit: non-stop

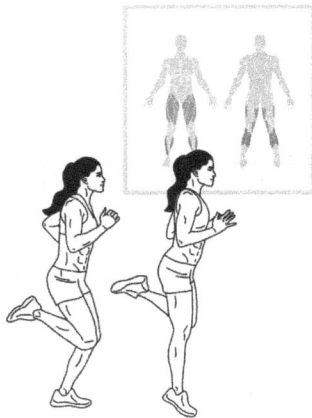

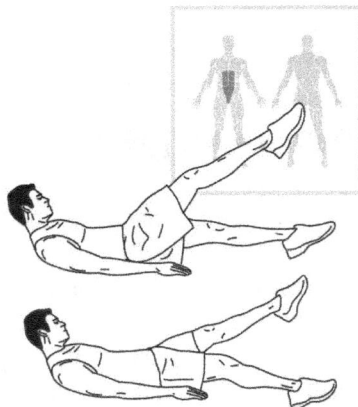

314

2 Minutes Flutter Kicks

Set a timer and do flutter kicks as
fast as you can for 2 minutes in total.
Split into manageable sets.

Extra Credit: non-stop

315

25 Up & Down Planks

Lower yourself from a plank into an elbow plank - 25 times in total. All the way down and all the way up is 1 rep. Split into manageable sets.

Extra Credit: in one go, keep the plank

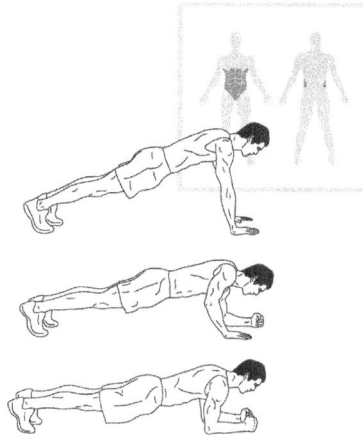

316

100 Jumping Jacks

Do jumping jacks until you hit 100 in total. Split into manageable sets.

Extra Credit: in one go

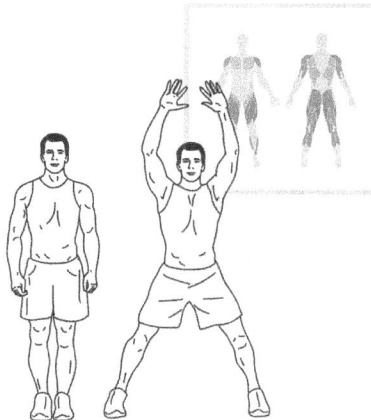

20 Cross Tricep Extensions

Get into a plank position, hands crossed over each other. Lower yourself down until your elbows touch the floor = 20 times in total. Split into manageable sets.

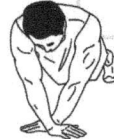

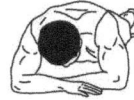

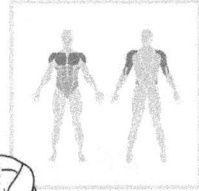

Extra Credit: in one go

50 Sitting Twists

Sit down on the floor or a sofa and do sitting twists, as illustrated - 50 in total. Split into manageable sets.

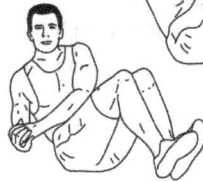

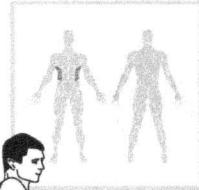

Extra Credit: in one go

319

50 Bridge Taps

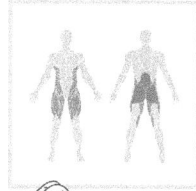

Lie down, raise your hips up and tap the floor over your head. Repeat 50 times in total. Split into manageable sets.

Extra Credit: in one go

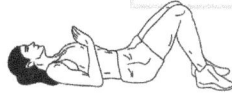
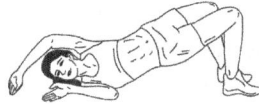

320

50 Balance Side Lunges

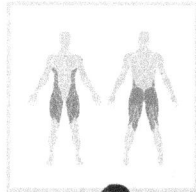

Raise your arms and one knee up. Step to the side into a lunge - 50 times in total. Split into manageable sets.

Extra Credit: in one go,

keep arms up

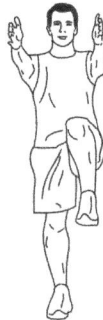
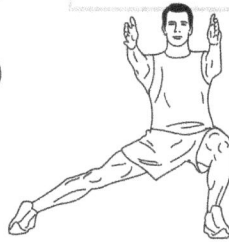

2 Minutes Half Bow

Set a timer and raise your arms
fingers pointing up. Bend your
elbows so your fingers point forward,
as illustrated - for 2 minutes in total.
Split into manageable sets.

Extra Credit: non-stop

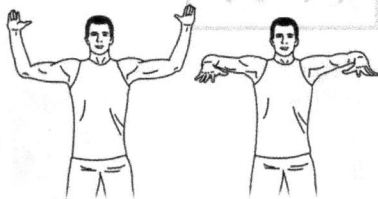

40 Windshield Wipers

Lie down on the floor or a bed, raise
your legs up at 90 degrees. Tilt them
to the left and then tilt them to the
right (= 2 reps) 40 times in total.

Extra Credit: in one go

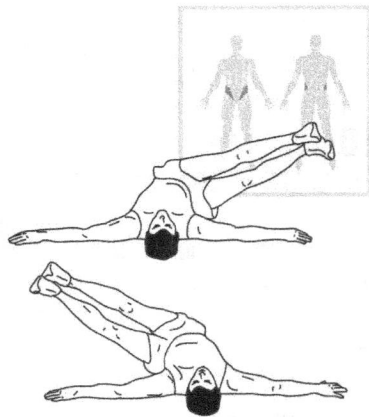

323

3 Minutes Side Splits

Set a timer and hold side splits (go as low as you can) for 3 minutes in total. Split into manageable sets.

Extra Credit: in one go

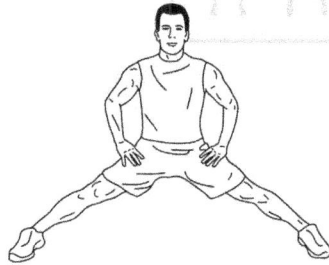

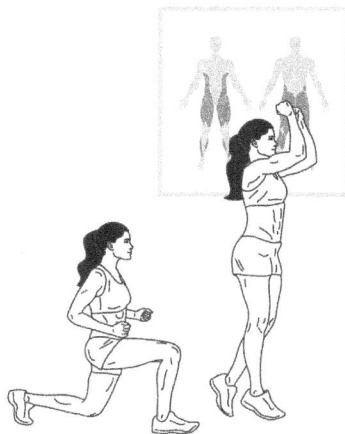

324

40 Jumping Lunges

Jump up and land into a lunge, try to jump as high as you can each time. Complete 20 reps on one side, then 20 reps on the other side = 40 times in total. Split into manageable sets.

Extra Credit: in one go

325

60 Knee Rolls

Lie down, knees bent as illustrated.
Roll them from side to side, until they
touch the floor - 60 times in total.
Split into manageable sets.

Extra Credit: in one go

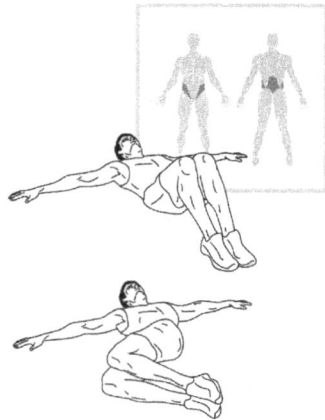

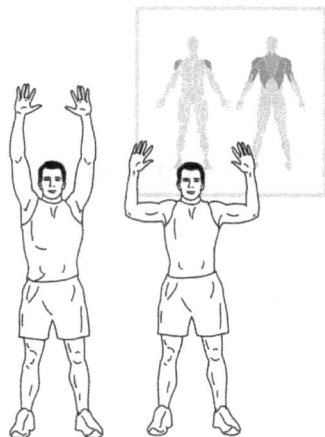

326

150 W-Arm Extensions

Raise your arms up and then lower
them down until your elbows are at
shoulder level - as illustrated. Repeat
150 times in total. Split into manageable sets.

Extra Credit: in one go

327

60 Squat Hold
Side Bends

Lower yourself into a squat and place your arms behind your head, as illustrated. Bend to the side and reach with your elbow to your knee - 60 times in total. Split into manageable sets.

Extra Credit: in one go

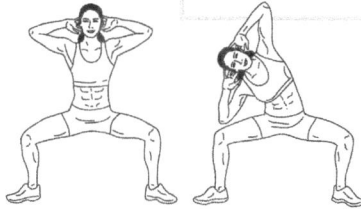

328

50 Half Shrimp Squats

Stand on one leg and grab the other one as illustrated and do squats - 40 in total. Split into manageable sets.

Extra Credit: 25 / 25, in one go

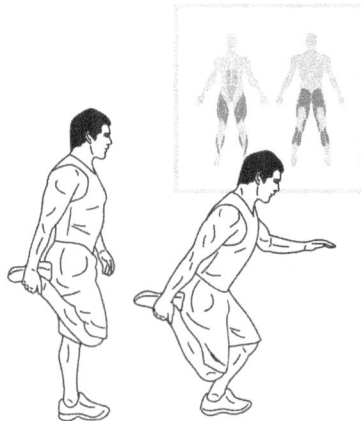

60 Seconds Star Plank

Get into a plank position, slide your arms and legs as far apart as you can and hold it for 60 seconds in total. Split into manageable sets.

Extra Credit: non-stop, keep the plank

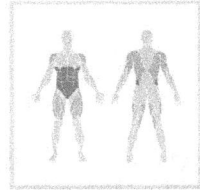

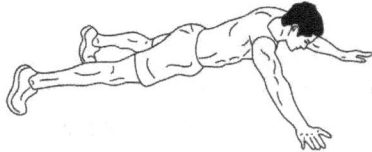

3 Minutes Raised Arm Circles

Set a timer, raise your arms up shoulder height and rotate them for 3minutes in total. Split into manageable sets.

Extra Credit: non-stop

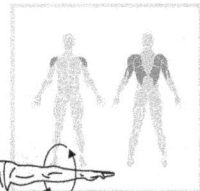

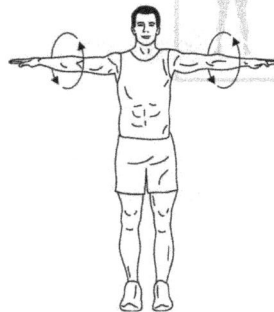

331

200 Standing Shoulder Taps

Tap your shoulders and raise your arms up reaching for the ceiling - 200 times in total. Split into manageable sets.

Extra Credit: in one go

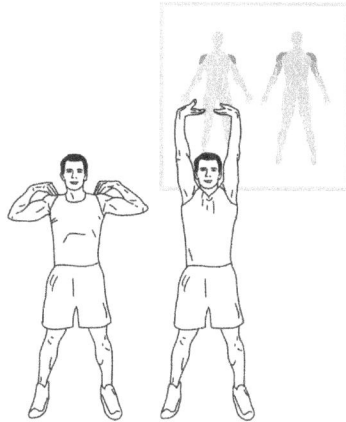

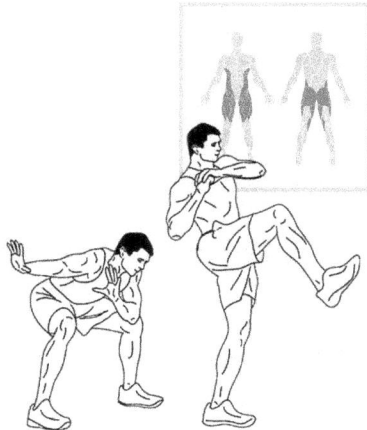

332

60 Squat Step-Ups

Squat and step up, as illustrated until you hit 30 reps, change sides and do another 30; 60 in total. Split into manageable sets.

Extra Credit: in one go

200 Uppercuts

Throw uppercuts until you hit 100.
Switch sides and throw another 100;
100 uppercuts in total . Split into
manageable sets.

Extra Credit: in one go

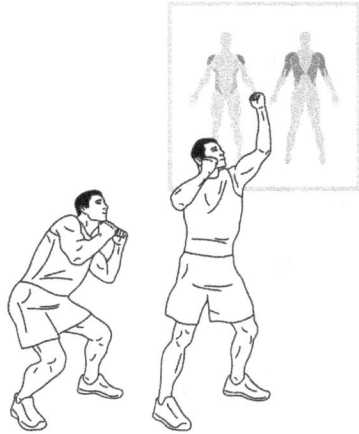

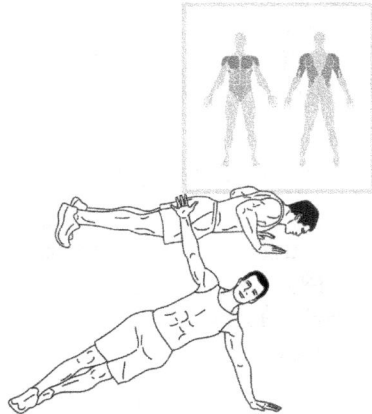

40 Push-Up
With Rotations

Get on the floor and lower yourself
into a push-up, come up and turn
into a side plank - 40 times in total;
split into manageable sets.

Extra Credit: in one go

335

2 Minutes Half Jacks

Set a timer and do half jacks for 2 minutes in total. Split into manageable sets.

Extra Credit: non-stop

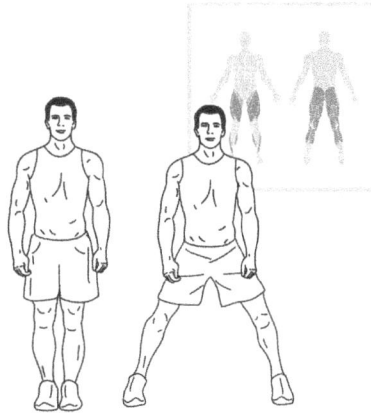

336

25 Basic Burpees With a Jump

Do basic burpees with a jump (no push-up) as fast as you can until you hit 25 in total. Split into manageable sets.

Extra Credit: in one go

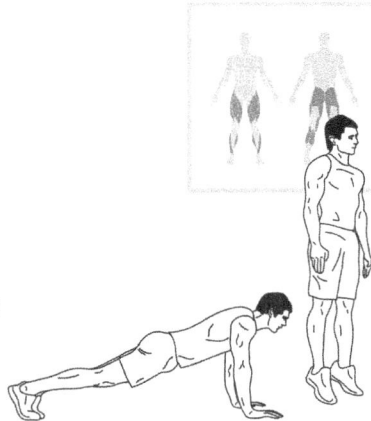

337

120 Side Leg Raises

Raise your right leg to your side
at 90 degrees until you hit 60 reps;
change legs and do another 60,
100 in total. You can hold on to
something.

Extra Credit: 60/60 in one go

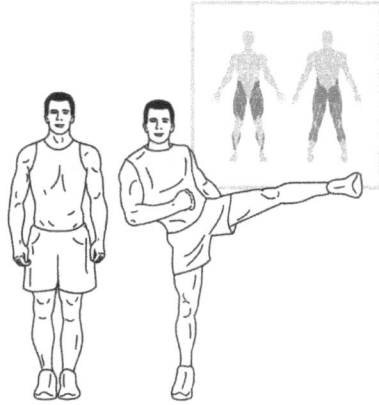

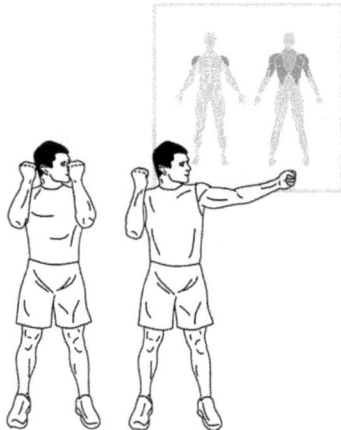

338

300 Backfists

Throw backfists to the right until
you hit 150, change sides and throw
backfists to the left - another 150;
300 times in total. Split into manageable sets.

Extra Credit: in one go

339

30 Push-Up + Jab + Cross

Drop into a push-up then jump up and throw a jab followed up by a cross. Repeat until you hit 30 in total. Split into manageable sets.

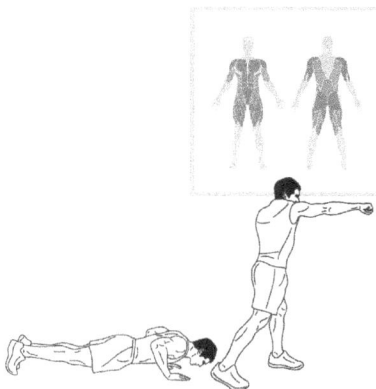

Extra Credit: in one go

340

140 Climbers

Get down into a plank. Begin to climb on the spot, as fast as you can, until you hit 140 reps in total (70 per leg). Split into manageable sets.

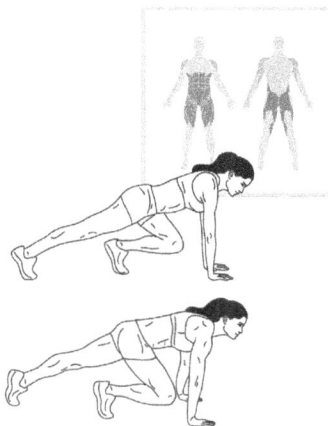

Extra Credit: in one go

50 Raised Leg Crunches

Lie down and raise your legs off the floor. Keep your legs up and do crunches until you hit 50 in total. Split into manageable sets.

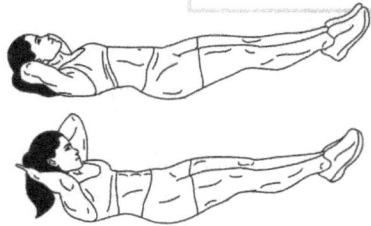

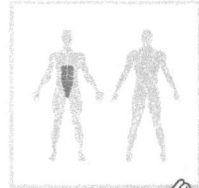

Extra Credit: in one go , keep legs up

100 Seal Jacks

Start with your arms raised to your sides, legs wide then jump in, bringing your hands together. Repeat 100 times in total.

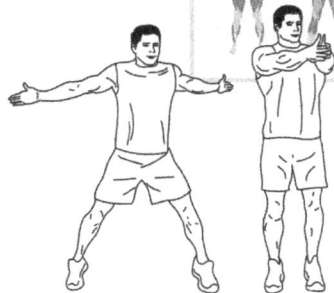

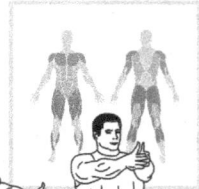

Extra Credit: in one go

40 Butt-Ups

Lie down on the floor, knees in.
Extend your legs towards the ceiling.
Repeat 40 times in total. Split into
manageable sets.

Extra Credit: in one go

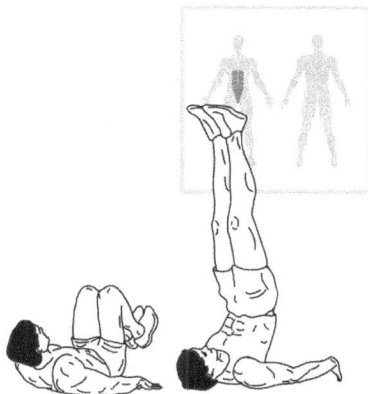

3 Minutes Tree Pose

Hold the Tree Pose (as illustrated) for
90 seconds in one go, change sides
and hold it for another 90 seconds.

Extra Credit: in one go, keep balance

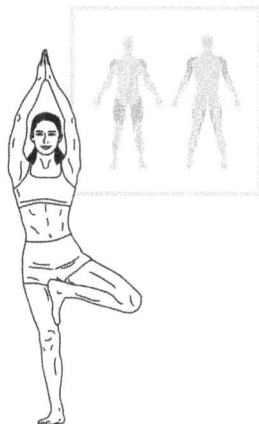

345

25 Plank Walk-Outs

Walk out into a plank, as illustrated, until you hit 25 in total. Split into manageable sets.

Extra Credit: in one go

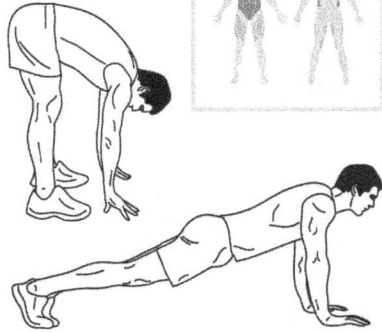

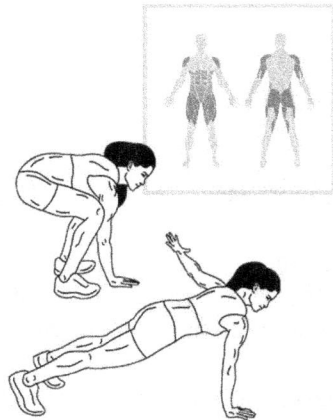

346

20 Single Arm Plank Jump-Ins

Get into a one-armed plank position - jump in and then back out 20 times in total (10 each arm); Split into manageable sets.

Extra Credit: in one go

347

50 Reverse Angels

Lie on the floor face down, arms extended in front of you. Bring your arms to your sides as illustrated 50 times in total. Split in to manageable sets.

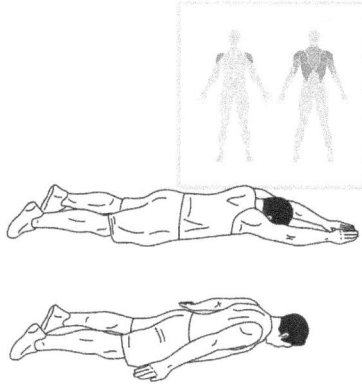

Extra Credit: in one go

348

50 Infinity Circles

Raise your leg to the side, waist height and draw infinity symbol in the air - 50 in total, 25 each leg. Split into manageable sets.

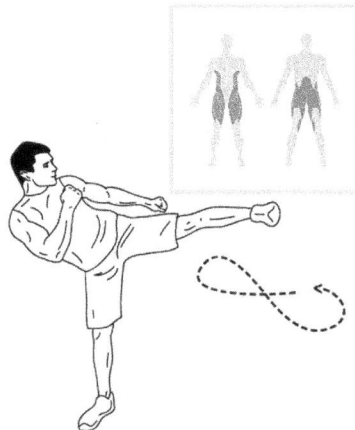

Extra Credit: in one go

40 Full Bridges

Sit down on the floor as illustrated and raise your hips up as high as you can - 40 times in total. Split into manageable sets.

Extra Credit: in one go

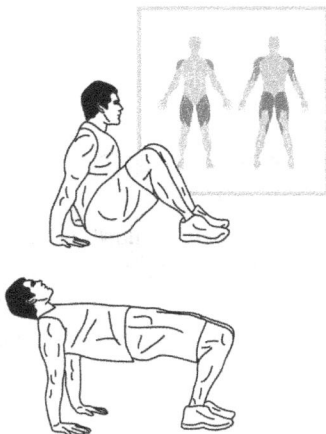

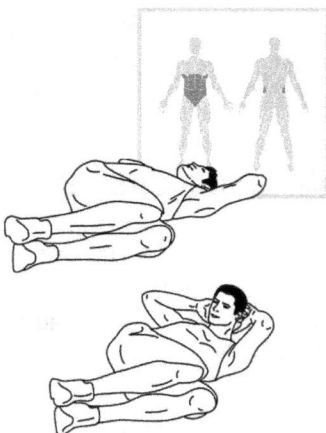

50 Folded Crunches

Lie down on the floor and fold your legs to the side as illustrated. Do crunches - 50 in total, 25 per side. Split into manageable sets.

Extra Credit: in one go

20 Jump Knee Tucks

Jump up bringing your knees to your chest - 20 times in total.
Split into manageable sets.

Extra Credit: in one go

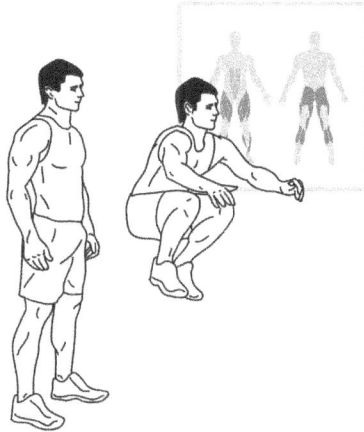

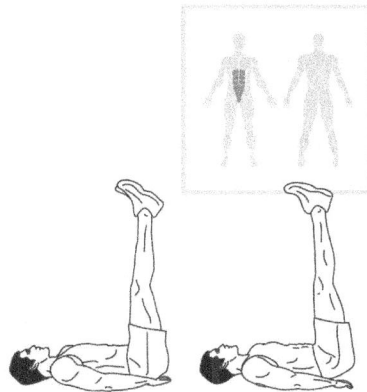

50 Pulse Ups

Lie down, raise your legs up at a 90 degrees angle and lift your hips off the floor slightly. Pulse up and down as illustrated 50 times in total.

Extra Credit: in one go

353

4 Minutes March Steps

Set a timer and do march steps
(march on the spot) for 4 minutes in
total. Split into manageable sets.

Extra Credit: non-stop

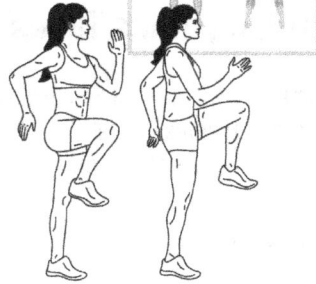

354

4 Minutes Leg Raise
Hold

Lie down on the floor on your side
and raise your leg at about 30 degrees - as illustrated. Hold it up for 4
minutes in total, 2 minutes per side.
Split into manageable sets.

Extra Credit: in one go

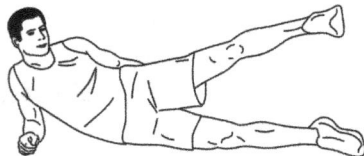

355

4 Minutes Meditation

Set a timer and meditate for
4 minutes in total. Relax. Keep cool.
Breathe.

Extra Credit: in one go

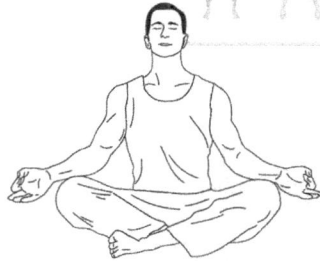

356

4 Minutes Chest Squeeze

Stand upright with both arms out
in front of you, bent at a 90 degree
angle. Lock your hands together and
squeeze as hard as you can. Hold the
contraction for 4 minutes in total.

Extra Credit: non-stop

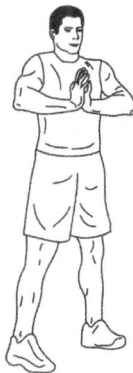

357

40 Raised Leg Circles

Get down on the floor and raise your legs at roughly 45 degrees. "Draw" circles in the air - 40 in total. Split into manageable sets.

Extra Credit: in one go

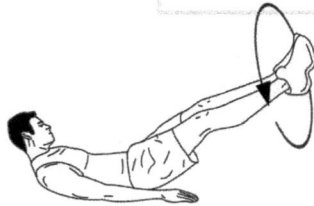

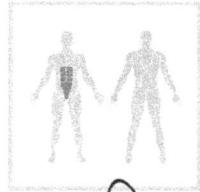

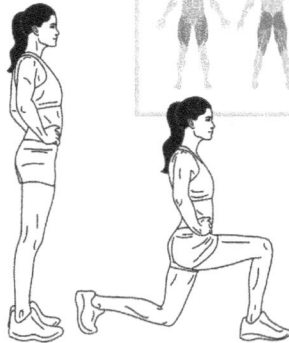

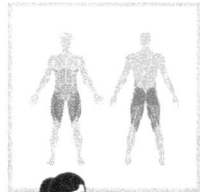

358

50 Forward Lunges

Step into a forward lunge 50 times in total. Split into manageable sets.

Extra Credit: in one go

30 Raised Leg Push-Ups

Get into a plank position and raise your left leg, lower yourself down and then push yourself up - 30 times in total. Switch legs every time. Split into manageable sets.

Extra Credit: in one go

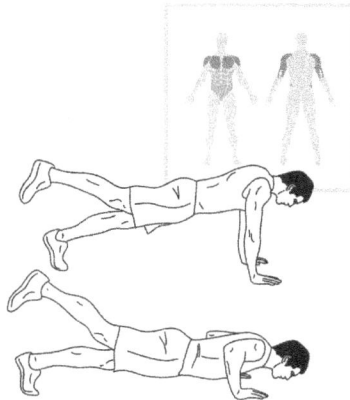

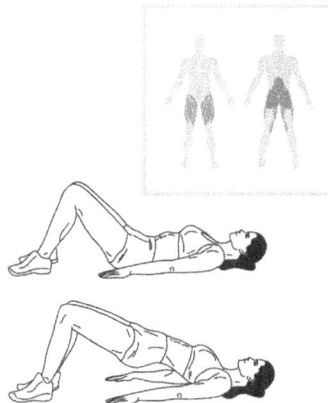

50 Bridges

Lie down, knees bent as illustrated and raise your hips off the floor = 50 times in total. Split into manageable sets.

Extra Credit: in one go

2 Minutes High Knees

Set a timer and do high knees (sprint on the spot) for 2 minutes in total. Split into manageable sets.

Extra Credit: non-stop

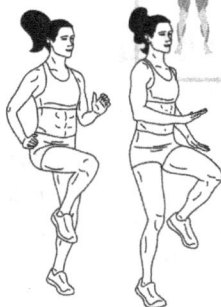

4 Minutes Wall-Sit

Set a timer and sit against the wall as illustrated. Hold it for 4 minutes in total. Split into manageable sets.

Extra Credit: in one go

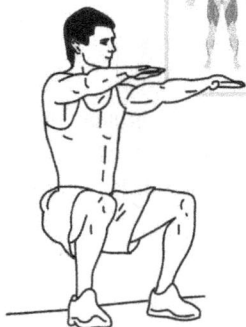

363

3 Minutes Clench / Unclench

Set a timer then clench and unclench your hands as fast as you can for 3 minutes in total. Split into manageable sets.

Extra Credit: non-stop

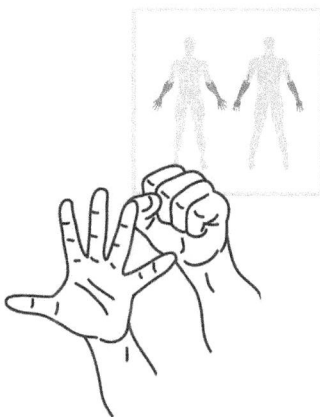

364

50 Push-Ups

Get into a plank position and do a push-up until you hit 30 in total. Split into manageable sets.

Extra Credit: in one go

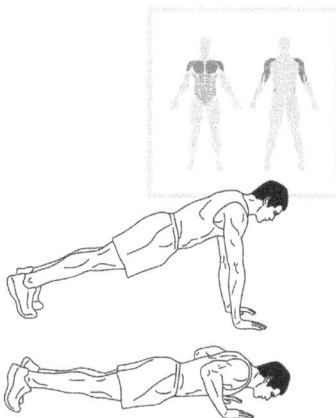

50 Sit-Ups

Lie down on the floor and do sit-ups until you hit 50 in total. Split into manageable sets.

Extra Credit: in one go

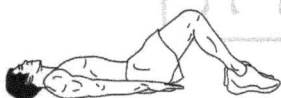

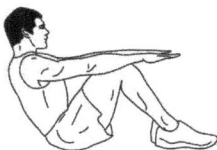

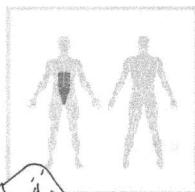

Fitness is a journey, not a destination.
Darebee Project

Thank you!

Thank you for purchasing 365 Daily Dares: Micro-Fitness for Everyone, DAREBEE project print edition. DAREBEE is a non-profit global fitness resource dedicated to making fitness accessible for everyone, no matter their circumstances. The project is supported exclusively via user donations and paperback royalties.

After printing costs and store fees every book developed by the DAREBEE project makes $1 and it goes directly into our project maintenance and development fund.

Each sale helps us keep the DAREBEE resource growing, maintain it and keep it up. Thank you for making a difference in its future!

Other books in this series include:

- 100 No-Equipment Workouts Vol 1.
- 100 No-Equipment Workouts Vol 2.
- 100 No-Equipment Workouts Vol 3.
- 100 Office Workouts
- 100 HIIT Workouts
- Pocket Workouts: 100 no-equipment workouts
- ABS 100 Workouts: Visual Easy-To-Follow ABS Exercise Routines for All Fitness Levels

www.ingramcontent.com/pod-product-compliance
Lightning Source LLC
Chambersburg PA
CBHW070838300326
41935CB00038B/1111